THIS BOOK CAN RAISE YOUR SCORE EVEN MORE!

You've bought this book because you're ready to prepare on your own. But what happens if you have a question? What if you need more help? Send back this card.

CALL US

On Monday through Friday nights, give us a call at **(800) 2-TEST-HI** between 6-11pm EST. Our instructors will be there to answer any questions you may have. It costs $1 per minute, in ten minute increments, and you'll pay ONLY for the time you're being tutored.

ACCESS US

It's even easier to ask a question by computer. On America Online and eWorld, you'll find us at *"The Princeton Review"*. On the Web, we're *www.review.com*. Or email us at *info@review.com*. We'll try to get you an answer within a day, at no fee.

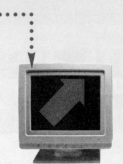

BUT FIRST, SEND BACK THIS CARD!

To use our phone and online support, just fill out this card and send it back now, or fax it to us at (212) 874-0775.

Your I.D. No. is

96-10326924

WHAT DO YOU WANT? (CHECK ALL THAT APPLY)

☐ PLEASE ACTIVATE MY **ID** NUMBER FOR PHONE AND ONLINE SUPPORT (SEE STUB FOR DETAILS OF SUPPORT PROGRAM).

☐ PLEASE SEND ME INFORMATION ABOUT PRINCETON REVIEW COURSES.

☐ PLEASE SEND ME INFORMATION ABOUT PAYING FOR SCHOOL (INCLUDING A STUDENT LOAN APPLICATION/INFORMATION).

96-10326924

Name: _____

Address: _____

City: _____ State:_____ Zip: _____

Phone: _____ E-mail Address: _____

Is that address ☐ School ☐ Work ☐ Home

School: _____ Graduation Year: _____

What test are you taking? _____

When do you plan to take it?_____

How did you hear about The Princeton Review? _____

Where did you buy this book (bookstore & city)? _____

What other preparation will you be doing for the test?_____

Other books in The Princeton Review Series

Cracking the New SAT and PSAT
Cracking the New SAT and PSAT with Sample Tests on Computer Disk
Cracking the ACT
Cracking the ACT with Sample Tests on Computer Disk
Cracking the LSAT
Cracking the LSAT with Sample Tests on Computer Disk
Cracking the GRE
Cracking the GRE with Sample Tests on Computer Disk
Cracking the GRE Psychology Test
Cracking the GMAT
Cracking the GMAT with Sample Tests on Computer Disk
Cracking the MCAT with Sample Tests on Computer Disk
Cracking the SAT II: Biology Subject Test
Cracking the SAT II: Chemistry Subject Test
Cracking the SAT II: English
Cracking the SAT II: French Subject Test
Cracking the SAT II: History Subject Tests
Cracking the SAT II: Math Subject Tests
Cracking the SAT II: Physics Subject Test
Cracking the SAT II: Spanish Subject Test
Cracking the TOEFL with audiocassette
How to Survive Without Your Parents' Money
Grammar Smart
Math Smart
Reading Smart
Study Smart
Writing Smart
Student Access Guide to America's Top 100 Internships
Student Access Guide to College Admissions
Student Access Guide to the Best Business Schools
Student Access Guide to the Best Law Schools
Student Access Guide to the Best Medical Schools
Student Access Guide to Paying for College
Student Access Guide to the Best 306 Colleges
Student Access Guide to Visiting College Campuses
Trashproof Resumes
Word Smart: Building an Educated Vocabulary
Word Smart II: How to Build a More Educated Vocabulary

Also available on cassette from Living Language

Grammar Smart
Word Smart
Word Smart II

THE PRINCETON REVIEW

CRACKING THE MCAT

BY THEODORE SILVER, M.D., AND THE
STAFF OF THE PRINCETON REVIEW

1996 EDITION

Random House, Inc.
New York 1995

ISBN: 0-679-76272-8

ISSN: 1067-2184

Manufactured in the United States of America

9 8 7 6 5 4 3 2

First 1996 Edition

CONTENTS

PART I

Orientation

INTRODUCTION

In April 1991 the Association of American Medical Colleges first administered its newly revised MCAT. Three months *earlier* (after two years of preparation), The Princeton Review opened its MCAT preparatory course nationwide, complete with four simulated MCATs. At The Princeton Review, we make it our business to know what standardized-test makers are up to, and that's one reason our courses consistently raise scores.

If you're preparing to take the MCAT, start with this book. It will assess your present ability as an MCAT candidate and set you moving on the road to a high score.

HOW THIS BOOK IS ORGANIZED

PART ONE *describes the MCAT* and tells you how to prepare.

PART TWO presents a *full-length simulated MCAT* with answer key and scoring grid.

PART THREE *explains the answers* to the simulated test that appears in Part Two. For every question, we tell you why a particular answer is right and why the others are wrong, so that you can understand your errors and start to correct them. For each of the writing problems, we provide a sample essay written according to The Princeton Review MCAT Essay Formula.

You'll get the most from this book if you pursue its three parts fully and *in their appropriate order*. Read Part One. Take the test provided in Part Two. Score yourself. Then identify your errors, strengths, and weaknesses by reading the explanations provided in Part Three.

PREPARING FOR THE MCAT / WHAT IS THE MCAT?

The MCAT (**M**edical **C**ollege **A**dmissions **T**est) is a seven-hour test that American medical schools use to admit and reject their applicants. If you're planning on attending medical school, you *have* to take the MCAT. It determines where you go—or whether you go at all.

WHO PRODUCES THE MCAT?

The MCAT is officially produced by a group called the Association of American Medical Colleges (AAMC). AAMC is supposed to be responsible for the MCAT. In exercising this responsibility it contracts with other people and testing companies who actually write and administer the test. Since 1991, when the "revised MCAT" was first introduced, AAMC seems to have had some trouble finding people and companies with which it's happy. In 1991 the test was written and administered by American College Testing (ACT) of Iowa. By 1993 it turned over the job of administering the test to Educational Testing Services of New Jersey. Now, for administration of the MCAT, AAMC has gone back to ACT of Iowa, which maintains an office called the MCAT Program Office in Iowa City.

WHAT'S THE MCAT LIKE, AND HOW MANY QUESTIONS DOES IT HAVE?

The MCAT has one component called Scientific Reasoning, another called Verbal Reasoning, and a third that requires you to write two essays.

SCIENTIFIC REASONING

The MCAT's scientific reasoning component is divided into two sections: "Physical Sciences" and "Biological Sciences." Physical Sciences means physics and inorganic chemistry. Biological Sciences means biology and organic chemistry.

The physical science section presents ten to eleven reading passages, each pertaining to physics or inorganic chemistry. Every passage is followed by six to ten multiple-choice questions that supposedly concern the passage and the relevant science.

In addition, the physical science section presents ten to fifteen questions that *don't* relate to passages. We call these questions "freestanding." Altogether the physical science section has about seventy-five questions, and you must answer them in one hour and forty minutes.

The biological science section is similarly structured. You get ten to eleven reading passages, each pertaining to biology and/or organic chemistry. For each passage there are six to nine multiple-choice questions. The section also features ten to fifteen freestanding items.

Like the physical science section, the biological science section presents about seventy-five questions that you must answer in one hour and forty minutes.

VERBAL REASONING

On its surface, the MCAT's verbal reasoning section resembles reading comprehension tests you've taken in the past. You're given ten or eleven passages, and on each passage you're asked five to seven questions. The passages concern the natural sciences, social sciences, and humanities. The total number of questions is sixty-five, and you must answer them in one hour and twenty-five minutes.

ESSAYS

The MCAT features two writing exercises. Each one presents you with a short statement and asks you to write an essay about it. For your first essay you might be given a statement like this:

"A government cannot enforce a law if its citizens oppose it."

And then be instructed to:

Write a unified essay in which you perform the following tasks. Explain what you think the above statement means. Describe a specific situation in which you believe a government can enforce a law if its citizens oppose it. Discuss what you think determines whether a government can enforce a law that the citizens oppose.

For your second essay you might be given a statement like this:
"No false statement can live indefinitely."

Once again, you'd be told to:

Write a unified essay in which you perform the following tasks. Explain what you think the above statement means. Describe a specific situation in which you believe a false statement can live indefinitely. Discuss what you think determines whether a false statement can or cannot live indefinitely.

You're allowed thirty minutes to write each essay.

In all, the MCAT features about 30 reading passages, 219 questions, and 2 essays. The total testing time is 7 hours (including an hour for lunch).

HOW IS THE MCAT SCORED?

Every MCAT candidate gets four scores:

- one for verbal reasoning

- one for physical science

- one for biological sciences

- one for the two writing samples combined

The verbal and scientific sections are scored on a scale of one to fifteen, on which one is low and fifteen is high. Scores of ten or above ("double-digit scores") are very good. The writing sample is scored on a scale of J–T, on which J is low and T is high.

Here's a table that shows you how the MCAT is designed and scored.

The MCAT			
Section	Question	Time	Score
Verbal Reasoning	65	85 minutes	1–15
Physical Sciences	77	100 minutes	1–15
Essay Writing	2	60 minutes	J–T
Biological Sciences	77	100 minutes	1–15

NOW, WHAT DOES THE MCAT *REALLY* TEST, AND HOW DO I PREPARE?

There are two answers to that question. AAMC says that the MCAT is just what it claims to be: a test of scientific reasoning, verbal reasoning, and writing ability. AAMC says you should prepare for the science sections by reviewing your college notebooks. It tells you to prepare for the verbal reasoning and writing sections by buying the sample questions and materials it offers for sale.

We at The Princeton Review have a different answer. We know the MCAT. We've taken it apart bit by bit, piece by piece, and shred by shred. We've studied it backward, forward, upside down, and inside out. We know what it tests and what it doesn't test, and we can tell you this:

- The MCAT does *not* test "reasoning"—verbal, scientific, or any other kind.
- Your college notes will not help you achieve a high score.

In order to prepare for the MCAT, you must appreciate the difference between studying *science* and studying *science for the MCAT*. You must review the premedical sciences in a way that is systematically tailored *to the test*. Furthermore, you must study MCAT questions themselves. You should be "wise" to their design and schooled in *techniques* that systematically lead to correct answers.

AAMC doesn't tell you these things. We do. So don't bother reviewing your college notes (as if you still had them) and don't prepare for a test of "reasoning."

AAMC's advice won't help you, ours will.

WAIT A SECOND. AAMC *PRODUCES* THE MCAT. SHOULDN'T I LISTEN TO THEM BEFORE I LISTEN TO YOU?

Good question. The answer is no. AAMC isn't on your side. It's not concerned with you, your score, or your future. AAMC is interested in *promoting the MCAT*. Every year it collects nearly $6 million by charging $150 per test to each of approximately 40,000 students. In order to continue collecting that money, AAMC must keep the medical schools believing that the MCAT is worthy of their attention so that the schools, in turn, will continue to require the MCAT of their applicants.

In other words, AAMC doesn't necessarily *want* you to do well on the MCAT. Too many high scores would make the test seem easy, and that would impair the MCAT's credibility. AAMC wants some test takers to get *low* scores. Low scores make the test look hard, and that's *good* for its credibility.

AAMC has no interest in helping you achieve a high score. It's the AAMC's business to peddle their test. *Our* business, on the other hand, is to raise your score. When we give you advice, that's our *only* concern.

SHOULD I BUY THE PRACTICE MATERIALS THAT AAMC SELLS?

Yes, you probably should. For a total of $36, AAMC will sell you two full-length MCATs and two booklets containing additional MCAT-like passages and questions. The materials do *not* include explanatory answers or a scoring grid (which allows you to calculate your scores on the one-to-fifteen scale). Nonetheless, the materials are worth having. To order them, write to:

AAMC
2450 N Street, N.W.
Washington, DC 20037

Enclose a check for $36 and a very short letter requesting:

(1) The MCAT Student Manual with Practice Test I
(2) MCAT Practice Test II with Practice Item Booklets

You might wish, instead, to call AAMC at 202-828-0416.

AAMC's materials are useful, but, as we said before, their *advice* is not. When it comes to advice about the MCAT, listen to people who are on *your* side. In other words, listen to *us*.

OKAY, I'M LISTENING. HOW *SHOULD* I PREPARE?

Naturally, you have to study physics, chemistry, biology, reading, and writing. But it's important that you approach all of these subjects in a way that's especially *tailored to the MCAT.* You must learn how MCAT questions are structured and how to select correct answers by *thinking like the test writers*.

Let's think first about science. MCAT test writers have a way of using a few simple principles to write a large variety of seemingly difficult questions. These questions are easy to answer if you understand the simple principles on which they're built.

HERE'S AN EXAMPLE: THE PRINCIPLE OF EQUILIBRIUM

Look at this physical science passage and the question that follows.

Passage I

Coal, a major source of energy, can be converted from its solid, raw form to a gaseous form of fuel. This is accomplished by the *water gas reaction* as shown below:

$$C(s) + H_2O(g) \rightleftharpoons CO(g) + H_2(g)$$

Solid carbon is reacted with steam to produce a mixture of carbon monoxide and hydrogen gas. This mixture is what is called "water gas." Water gas is highly combustible. The following table lists the standard heats of formation and free energies of formation of each of the four compounds in the water gas reaction.

	ΔH_f°(KJ/mol)	ΔG_f°(KJ/mol)
$CO(g)$	−110.5	−137.3
$H_2(g)$	0.0	0.0
$C(s)$	0.0	0.0
$H_2O(g)$	−241.8	−228.6

1. Assume a chemist initiates the water gas reaction and then, as the reaction proceeds, invests the surroundings with an extraordinarily high concentration of carbon monoxide. Among the following, which would most likely result?

    I. Water gas will undergo complete and immediate combustion.
    II. Ambient steam concentration will decrease.
    III. Ambient hydrogen concentration will decrease.

    A. I only
    B. III only
    C. I and II only
    D. I and III only

To the student who approaches the MCAT *strategically,* this question is easy. She knows, first of all, that she can answer it *without reading the passage.* She need only:

(1) look at the "water gas reaction" and

(2) understand the principle of equilibrium.

LET'S UNDERSTAND EQUILIBRIUM

Look at this equilibrium equation.

$$A + B \rightleftharpoons C + D$$

On the left side of the equilibrium equation we find A and B. On the right side we find C and D. A and B act together to produce C and D. C and D, meanwhile, act together to produce A and B.

$$A + B \longrightarrow C + D$$
$$A + B \longleftarrow C + D$$

If we add more A to the solution, we're going to get *more* C and D. That's true even if we don't add any more B. Adding more A, by itself, will increase the production of C and D (until we've used up all of the B, at which point adding more A won't increase the production of C and D).

$$\overset{add\,A}{\searrow} A + B \longrightarrow {\uparrow}C + {\uparrow}D$$

If we add more B to the solution, we're also going to get more C and D. That's true even if we don't add any more A. Adding more B, by itself, will increase the production of C and D (until we've used up all of the A, at which point adding more B won't increase the production of C and D).

$$\overset{add\,B}{\searrow} A + B \longrightarrow {\uparrow}C + {\uparrow}D$$

Adding more A *and* B, of course, will also increase the production of C and D.

When we increase the production of C and D, we are "driving the equilibrium to the right." In other words, we're causing increased production of the stuff that's on the right side of the equilibrium equation.

Adding more C or more D to the system has an analogous but opposite effect. If we add more C, we'll increase the production of A and B unless and until we run out of D. If we add more D to the system we'll increase the production of A and B unless and until we run out of C.

THINK ABOUT IT THIS WAY

When you add more A or B to the system, you're making things kind of crowded on the left side of the equation. In order to relieve the crowding, the system decides to move over to the right. Similarly, if you add more C or D to the system, you're making things kind of crowded on the right. The system adjusts by moving to the left.

Now, let's think about this. We know that when we add either C or D, by itself, we get more of A and B. But when we add more C, by itself, what happens to the concentration of D? In other words, when we increase the concentration of a species on the right side of an equation, what happens to the concentration of the *other* species on the right side of the equation?

It goes down.

When we add more C to the system, there will be more collisions between C particles and D particles. That's how we form more A and B. Since we did not add any D to the system, the increased collisions among C and D particles and the increased production of A and B will tend to *reduce* the concentration of D.

In other words, adding more C to the system crowds things up on the right. In order to relieve themselves of the crowding, some C particles and D particles pack up and move over to the left (where they become A and B particles). So, the concentration of D goes down.

The overall concentration of C does *not* go down. The crowding began because we *added* C. It's true that some of the newly added C particles will get together with D and move to the left. But they won't *all* do that. After the equilibrium has shifted, there will be more C particles on the right than there were before we added any C. There will be fewer D particles on the right than there were before we began, and there will, of course, be more A and B particles on the left.

LOOK AGAIN AT THE "WATER GAS REACTION" AND ANSWER THE QUESTION

$$C(s) + H_2O(g) \rightleftharpoons CO(g) + H_2(g)$$

1. Assume a chemist initiates the water gas reaction and then, as the reaction proceeds, invests the surroundings with an extraordinarily high concentration of carbon monoxide. Among the following, which would most likely result?

    I. Water gas will undergo complete and immediate combustion.
    II. Ambient steam concentration will decrease.
    III. Ambient hydrogen gas concentration will decrease.

    A. I only
    B. III only
    C. I and II
    D. I and III

Choice B is correct. When the chemist exposes the equilibrium to high concentrations of CO, he is, in effect, adding CO to the right side of the equation. The right side gets "crowded," and the equilibrium shifts to the left. That means:

(1) the concentration of hydrogen gas *decreases*

(2) the concentration of steam (gaseous water) *increases*, and

(3) the concentration of solid carbon *increases*.

The equilibrium principle generates a variety of MCAT questions pertaining to inorganic chemistry, organic chemistry, and physics. It underlies *seemingly* complicated MCAT problems involving acids, bases, buffers, syntheses, degradations, kinetics, and thermodynamics. To make the questions seem especially unapproachable, the MCAT writers set them behind a veil of graphs, tables, and diagrams—often useless and irrelevant. You'll bypass such distractions and make your way easily to correct answers *if you see the questions for what they are*—simple applications of the equilibrium principle.

Equilibrium represents *only one* of the simple principles on which MCAT questions are built. There are *many others*. You'll raise your score if you know what they are and how they operate.

ARE THERE TECHNIQUES I SHOULD LEARN FOR THE VERBAL REASONING COMPONENT?

Yes, definitely. The MCAT's verbal reasoning section is susceptible to several systems and strategies. Here, for example, are two devices that help you eliminate wrong answer choices.

DEVICE # 1: *RECOGNIZE STATEMENTS IN THE EXTREME*

When it comes to the MCAT's verbal reasoning section, an answer choice that is immoderate or extreme is seldom correct. When an answer choice pivots on words like "never," "always," "invariably," "only," "total," "ideal," or "perfect," it's almost certainly wrong. In the MCAT world, very few things are *absolute*.

Without even reading a passage, consider this question:

1. The author's claim that "productivity is the soul of civilization" (line 15) introduces his argument that:

   A. economics is the only important aspect of civilized life.
   B. civilizations are built primarily on economic foundations.
   C. people should devote their energies to their own fortunes and not to the problems of others.
   D. human beings are totally dependent on one another for all of their needs.

Choice A is extreme, and you can be pretty sure it's wrong. The idea that economics is the "only" important aspect of civilized life is contrary to MCAT philosophy. Choice D features the words "totally" and "all." It, too, is extreme and almost certainly wrong.

Consider this question and eliminate the choices that are extreme.

2. The author believes that practicing psychiatrists:

   A. cannot possibly help patients unless they are completely objective.
   B. are hopelessly confused over the genesis of mental illness.
   C. are scientists notwithstanding the uncertainties that surround them.
   D. should for the time being treat mental disease in terms of environment.

Choices A and B are extreme. The phrases "cannot possibly," "completely objective," and "hopelessly confused" should tip you off.

DEVICE # 2: *RECOGNIZE STATEMENTS THAT AREN'T "NICE"*

An answer choice contrary to the kinds of ideas in which "nice people" believe should be eliminated. Consider, for example, these thoughts:

- Violent criminals should not be viewed as human beings.

- Freedom of religion is destructive to a society.

- Children should be encouraged not to make friends with other children whose backgrounds are different from their own.

- Teachers should resort to stern discipline in order to maintain their students' attention.

These ideas just aren't *nice*. They don't conform to progressive and "enlightened" thought. They're never going to be correct answer choices. With that in mind, consider these two questions. Eliminate

—extremes and

—statements that aren't "nice."

3. The author believes that patients with serious psychiatric disturbances:

   A. are entirely beyond the reach of even the most competent psychotherapists.
   B. may have internal vulnerabilities on which an adverse environment has acted.
   C. are usually to blame for their illnesses and do not deserve treatment.
   D. are not likely to be physically strong.

When you read Choice A, the word "entirely" should ring a warning bell. Choice A is *extreme,* and you should eliminate it.

Choice C isn't "nice." "Nice" people don't blame psychiatric patients for their own illnesses. Such a sentiment won't be a correct answer on the MCAT. Choice C should be eliminated.

4. The passage suggests that criminal attorneys will be most successful in helping their clients if they:

   A. endeavor to give those clients a sense of self-esteem.
   B. identify, personally, with the client's situation.
   C. never offer advice, and limit themselves entirely to asking questions.
   D. treat those clients not like human beings but like diseased organisms.

When you read Choice C the words "never" and "entirely" should trigger an alarm. Choice C is *extreme*. Eliminate it.

Choice D isn't "nice." "Nice" people think all clients should be treated as human beings. Choice D could not possibly be correct.

There are a great many strategies and techniques that lead you to correct answers on the MCAT's verbal reasoning section, and it's important that you use them.

ARE THERE STRATEGIES AND TECHNIQUES FOR THE *WRITING SAMPLE* TOO?

Yes. In order to score well on your MCAT essays it's important, first of all, to know how they're graded. An MCAT essay is normally read by two graders. Each grader spends around ninety seconds (that's right, ninety *seconds*) reading an essay. She then grades it "holistically." Holistic grading is *supposed* to mean that the reader does not make separate evaluations in terms of substance, organization, or grammar. Rather, she's supposed to keep all these criteria somewhere in her mind (for ninety seconds) and then assign a grade based on an overall "sense" of the essay's quality.

AS WE SAID, THAT'S WHAT HOLISTIC GRADING IS *SUPPOSED* TO MEAN

Unfortunately, holistic grading *really* means that MCAT readers won't be giving any serious attention to the quality of your writing or what you're trying to express. In ninety seconds they can't possibly do that. Instead, they'll be grading your essay *based on the impression it makes on them*.

So, writing an MCAT essay means writing something that, in ninety seconds, will *impress* the reader and make her think well of you.

That means you should:

- make your essay easy to read,

- at least give the *appearance* of careful organization, *and*

- use words and phrases that make you seem "wise, serious, and well read."

All of these objectives can be achieved by following an MCAT essay *formula*. Here, for example, is an MCAT essay that's written according to the formula we teach in The Princeton Review MCAT course.

Consider this statement:

A society that is well educated will necessarily be free.

Write a unified essay in which you perform the following tasks: Explain what you think the above statement means. Describe a specific situation in which a well-educated society might not be free. Discuss what you think determines whether or not a well-educated society is free.

Response

The statement indicates that developed intellects seek social and political freedom and, furthermore, that a totalitarian or tyrannical government will ultimately fail in the face of an informed and insightful public. (A similar thought is manifest in Victor Hugo's remark that "One can resist the invasion of armies but not the invasion of ideas.") Those who have honestly and openly explored humanity's intellectual insights and discoveries will likely have the wish and the means to establish free societies.

In order specifically to describe a situation in which the statement does not apply, one need only recognize that the words "educated" and "freedom" are inherently ambiguous. The statement pivots on these words, and its applicability depends on the meanings attached to them. As used in the statement, "education" is subject to interpretation. It might refer to broad knowledge and understanding of history, science, and the arts and letters. On the other hand, it might signify only *formal schooling,* and schools, to be sure, need not educate. The "education" that a given school affords depends on the objectives of those who select its curriculum.

The dictator's school will teach that which fosters reverence for the dictator: intolerance, chauvinism, self-aggrandizement, and fear. Lessons may be rigorous and discipline may be stern. Students are not likely, however, to emerge with the sort of open-minded inquisitiveness that demands political freedom. In that sense, then, "education" need not give rise to freedom.

The phrase "free society" also harbors ambiguity. To some it signifies a capitalistic economy akin to that which operates in the United States. Thus understood, a "free society" does not necessarily accompany an educated populace. The spread of knowledge and learning over this past century seems to have brought widening acceptance of egalitarian principles. That has led, in turn, to widespread socialization of western and eastern economies and to a significant *restriction* on what might be termed economic freedom.

Hence the pertinence of the statement depends in large measure on the meaning attached to its language. If "education" refers to a genuine exposure to humanity's intellectual achievements and "freedom" means social and political liberty, then the statement represents a meaningful comment. If, however, "education" means "school," and "freedom" signifies economic opportunity, the statement is not accurate.

Because this essay was written according to a carefully devised formula,

- it addresses all three of the assigned "tasks."

- it seems to be carefully conceived and well organized.

- its writer appears to be "serious" about life, learning, and language.

Those are the ingredients of a high-scoring MCAT essay.

WILL THIS BOOK GIVE ME EVERYTHING I NEED?

To be honest—probably not. Unless you're starting out as a top MCAT student, no *book* can fully prepare you for the MCAT—not this one or any other. If you're serious about earning a high MCAT score, you need a good teacher, powerful materials, personal contact, and *repeated opportunities to take simulated tests that are scored, analyzed, and returned.*

In The Princeton Review MCAT course, for example, students attend sixteen, $3\frac{1}{2}$ hour sessions over an eight-week period. Teachers are dynamic, and classes are small. Each student works his way through twelve hundred pages of carefully designed teaching materials and thousands of exercises. Students are privately tutored, and between meetings they telephone their teachers whenever they feel the need. Separate from their class sessions, students take four simulated MCATs. Each test is scored, analyzed, and returned within a few days so that teacher and students may subject it to thorough review. For fifty-six days our students eat, sleep, and dream the MCAT. Such are the elements of a high MCAT score, and *no book can possibly provide all of them*, regardless of the promises made on its cover.

BUT THIS BOOK IS THE PLACE TO BEGIN

Find out where you stand and what you need. Set aside a full day and *take the simulated MCAT in this book*. Treat it seriously and subject yourself rigorously to MCAT test conditions:

- Start early in the morning, and for the whole day consider yourself absolutely unavailable for anything or anyone else.

- For each section give yourself only as much time as the instructions allow.

- Take the ten-minute breaks as indicated and take a full sixty-minute lunch hour between the Physical Science and Writing Sample sections of the test.

When you've finished the test, score yourself. Use the scoring key on page 96, and derive your scores for Verbal Reasoning, Physical Sciences, and Biological Sciences. (You can't score the writing sample, but we definitely want you to complete that section of the test anyway.)

YES, THEN WHAT?

If both your verbal and science scores are *10 or above* you're in pretty good shape. Depending on your college grades and the medical school you want to attend, you might consider signing up for the MCAT without pursuing special preparation. Naturally, you should review any science that gives you trouble on our simulated test. Then, for a few weeks before you take the real test, sit down and address the sample tests and materials that AAMC provides. If that goes smoothly, take the MCAT as scheduled. You'll probably do well.

On the other hand, if your verbal and science scores are *9 or below,* you've got to raise them. That probably means you should consider a good MCAT course.

CHOOSING AN MCAT COURSE

Generally speaking, a *good* MCAT course will:

1. Provide you with teachers, teaching systems, and teaching materials that organize your work, maintain your attention, and monitor your progress day by day and week by week.

2. Thoroughly immerse you in physics, inorganic chemistry, organic chemistry, biology, reading, and writing—in a way that is strategically designed *for the MCAT.*

3. Show you, systematically, how MCAT questions are structured and teach you how to select correct answers quickly by thinking like the test writers.

4. Give you repeated opportunities to take simulated MCATs that are quickly scored and returned to you for thorough review. Anyone who tries to prepare for the MCAT without repeated MCAT test taking might as well prepare for a driver's road test without ever getting behind a steering wheel. Hands-on practice with simulated MCATs is essential to raising scores.

Any course that fails to offer these four features is useless, no matter how many papers, booklets, or tapes it provides.

LET'S BE MORE SPECIFIC

Think about science. Some MCAT courses offer you stacks of science outlines and summaries that seem to "cover everything." Such materials are cheap and easy to design because they're only condensed versions of the textbooks you already own. Ironically, these outlines and summaries are much harder to get through than the textbooks themselves. They give you incomplete, watered-down information, and they skip key steps in the explanation process. Most people find them frustrating and confusing. Even if you do get through them (which you won't), they can't help you much. They don't teach science *the way the MCAT tests it*.

Here, for instance, is a sample from an MCAT course we'll call Course X. Try reading it.

9.3.1.1: Human Respiratory Function

A. Anatomy of Respiratory System: Respiratory tract —nares, bronchi (left and right main stem and subdivisions), bronchioles, terminal bronchioles, alveolar sacs and alveolus (site of gas exchange, see below). Bronchial secretions moved by cilia and cough reflex (autonomic, vagal).

B. Inspiratory function: Lung and chest wall have static and dynamic properties. Elasticity permits influx and efflux of gas. Diaphragm contracts (involuntary function, phrenic nerve signal initiated in CNS: medullary respiratory center), creates negative intrapulmonary pressure. Air traverses respiratory tract.

Tidal volume = air normally inspired.
Total capacity = full expansion.
Vital capacity = full exhalation.
Functional residual capacity = gas remaining after exhalation
Residual volume = gas remaining after full exhalation.

- Resistance to air flow (inspiratory and expiratory) caused by airway caliber. Combined total cross-sectional area increases at deeper levels (bronchioles, alveoli).

- Asthma and Emphysema (Chronic Obstructive Pulmonary Disease) produced by loss of elastic tissue, reduced airway caliber.

The material you just read is junk. It couldn't possibly help you answer a single question on the MCAT. To begin with, it's incomprehensible. No Earthly creature could figure out what it's trying to teach about respiration unless he fully understood and remembered the subject *beforehand* (in which case he wouldn't need a course).

Second, even if Course X were understandable, it would be teaching the *wrong information*. The MCAT does require that you know something about respiration. You have to comprehend the structure of the respiratory tract and understand the dynamics of inspiration, expiration, and gas exchange. Course X doesn't help you do that. Instead, it presents a hodgepodge of facts, most of which have no bearing on the MCAT. The MCAT will never ask you the meaning of terms like "tidal volume," "total capacity," or "functional residual capacity." (If those terms should happen to appear on the MCAT, their meaning will be explained.)

NOW READ *THIS* MATERIAL ABOUT RESPIRATION:

Your Brain Thinks You Should Breathe

The signal to breathe originates in the medulla oblongata, which is part of the brain. As you might expect, the signal originates in a part of the medulla that is called the respiratory center. It travels to the diaphragm via a nerve, and that nerve is called the phrenic nerve.

The diaphragm is a muscle. When stimulated by the phrenic nerve, it contracts. Contraction of the diaphragm begins the process of breathing in, which is called inspiration.

249. ☐ **TRUE** ☐ **FALSE** The diaphragm is a muscle.

250. ☐ **TRUE** ☐ **FALSE** The diaphragm receives its signal to contract from the vagus nerve.

251. ☐ **TRUE** ☐ **FALSE** The diaphragm receives its signal to contract from the phrenic nerve.

252. With respect to human respiration, the signal that initiates inspiration arises in the:

   A. cerebral cortex.
   B. medulla oblongata.
   C. trachea.
   D. vagus nerve.

253. Which of the following correctly orders the sequence in which the listed structures act to produce inspiration?

    A. Phrenic nerve, diaphragm, medulla oblongata
    B. Diaphragm, phrenic nerve, medulla oblongata
    C. Phrenic nerve, medulla oblongata, diaphragm
    D. Medulla oblongata, phrenic nerve, diaphragm

Look at This Syringe

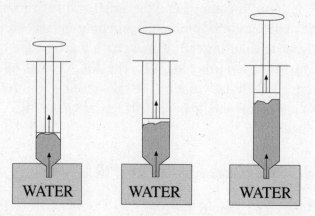

When the plunger rises, it creates negative pressure inside the cylinder. The negative pressure draws the water in, and the syringe fills.

Now, Look at the Diaphragm

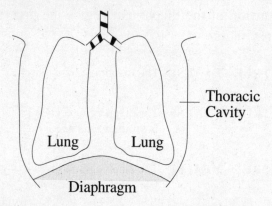

Before the diaphragm contracts, it is shaped like a dome. Then, when it does contract, it flattens out and creates empty space within the thoracic cavity. The empty space creates negative pressure. In order to fill the space and eliminate the negative pressure, the lungs expand.

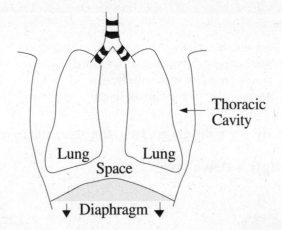

The Lungs Expand Even Though They Don't Want To

The lungs have a natural elasticity that tends to keep them from expanding. It's as though they had rubber bands around them "trying" to keep them closed. The negative pressure that arises when the diaphragm contracts causes the lungs to expand, even though they must "stretch" their rubber bands to do that.

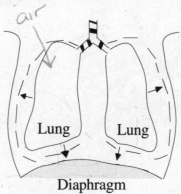

When the lungs do expand, they create a negative pressure inside themselves. In order to eliminate that negative pressure, air rushes into the lungs to fill the newly available space. That completes the process of inspiration.

254. ☐ **TRUE** ☐ **FALSE** During the process of inspiration, the lungs expand because the contraction of the diaphragm produces positive pressure in the thoracic cavity surrounding the lungs.

255. ☐ **TRUE** ☐ **FALSE** The pressure inside the lungs, at the moment they expand, is lower than the pressure in the atmosphere.

256. During the process of inspiration, air moves into the lungs in direct response to:

   A. negative pressure within the thoracic cavity.
   B. positive pressure within the thoracic cavity.
   C. positive pressure within the lungs.
   D. negative pressure within the lungs.

Now—how, exactly, does the air get from the atmosphere to the lungs?

By Climbing an Upside-Down Tree

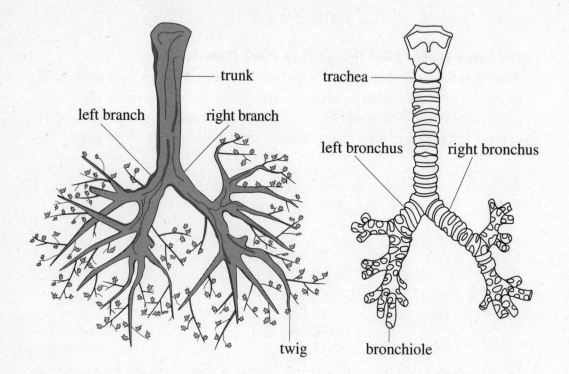

Does the Respiratory Tract Have Rings?

The trachea and bronchi have rings on their outside, and these rings are made of cartilage.

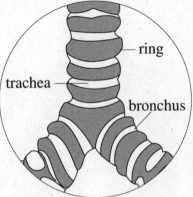

RESPIRATORY TRACT

The rings help keep the trachea and bronchi open.

How Does the Respiratory Tract Keep Itself Clean?

The respiratory tract begins with the nose. The nose cleans, warms, and moistens incoming air. Large particles are trapped in hairs lining the nostrils.

Particles that make it past the nose get stuck in mucus that lines the lower parts of the respiratory tree. Ciliated cells sweep the dirty mucus back out of the system. Very small particles can make it all the way to the alveoli, and these particles are eaten by phagocytic cells lining the alveoli.

257. ❐ TRUE ❐ FALSE Between the point where air enters at the nose and then settles in the alveoli, the human respiratory tract undergoes repeated branching.

258. ❐ TRUE ❐ FALSE Within the human respiratory tract, bronchi outnumber bronchioles, and bronchi outnumber alveoli.

259. Within the human respiratory tract, bronchi branch to form bronchioles, and bronchioles branch to terminate in:

A. bronchi.
B. the trachea.
C. alveoli.
D. the nose.

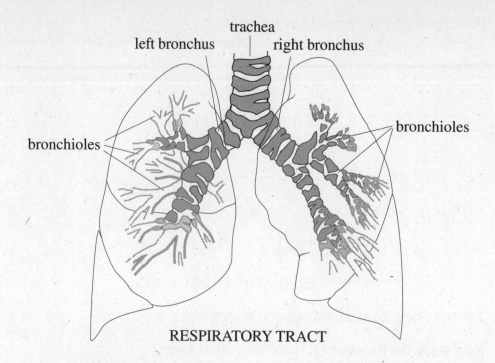

trachea

left bronchus   right bronchus

bronchioles   bronchioles

RESPIRATORY TRACT

The entire respiratory tract is like a tree turned upside down. First air enters the nose and flows into a trunk. The trunk is actually called the trachea. Next, the air reaches a "fork" in the trunk. These right and left branches are called bronchi. The bronchi themselves break up into smaller branches, and these smaller branches split several times more. The tiny twiglike branches are called bronchioles.

Does the Respiratory Tract Have Leaves?

No, but it does have things called alveoli. A little later we'll talk about what the alveoli do.

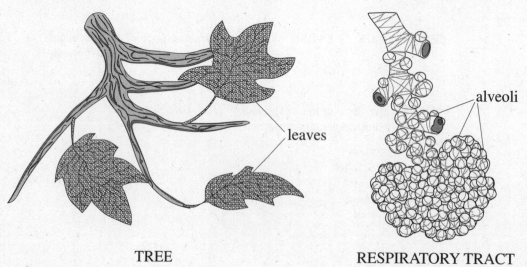

leaves

alveoli

TREE   RESPIRATORY TRACT

260. ☐ **TRUE** ☐ **FALSE** Within the human respiratory tract, rings surround the outside of the trachea and bronchi in order to help keep the airway open.

261. Within the human respiratory tract, the structure that cleans, warms, and moistens the air is:

  A. the bronchus.
  B. the trachea.
  C. the alveolus.
  D. the nose.

262. ☐ **TRUE** ☐ **FALSE** Mucus-covered ciliated cells prevent only the largest particles from reaching the alveoli.

The material you just read will raise your MCAT score. Its explanations are friendly, understandable, and coherent. They cover the substance you need for the MCAT, and they're likely to stay with you through the day you take the test. Furthermore, they include a multitude of pointed questions that maintain your attention and track your progress. *Together with a teacher's interactive review,* the material you just read will provide the knowledge you need to answer MCAT questions about respiration.

ENOUGH TALK—LET'S TAKE THE FIRST STEP

We've described the MCAT, and we've told you how to prepare for it. Now it's time to get started. Set aside a day and take the sample MCAT that's provided in Part Two of this book. Use the answer sheet provided at the back of the book. Time yourself according to the standard MCAT testing day:

Morning

Verbal Reasoning:	1 hour, 25 minutes
Break:	10 minutes
Physical Sciences:	1 hour, 40 minutes
Lunch:	1 hour

Afternoon

Writing Sample (I):	30 minutes
Writing Sample (II):	30 minutes
Break:	10 minutes
Biological Sciences:	1 hour, 40 minutes

After you've taken the test, score yourself. Then, over the next few days, evaluate your performance carefully by reading the explanatory answers provided in Part Three. They'll show you what you did right and what you did wrong. When you're all done you'll know just where you stand. You'll know where you're strong, you'll know where you're weak, and you'll be ready to plan your route toward a higher score.

From all of us at The Princeton Review: Good luck.

PART II

The Princeton Review MCAT Diagnostic Test

Verbal Reasoning

Time: 85 Minutes
Questions 1–65

VERBAL REASONING

DIRECTIONS: There are nine passages in the Verbal Reasoning test. Each passage is followed by several questions. After reading a passage, select the one best answer to each question. If you are not certain of an answer, eliminate the alternatives that you know to be incorrect and then select an answer from the remaining alternatives. Indicate your selection by blackening the corresponding circle on your answer sheet (DIAGNOSTIC TEST FORM).

Passage I (Questions 1–7)

The Michelson-Morley experiment of 1887 successfully demonstrated that if two beams of light were dispatched from a single observer standing on the Earth, one in the direction of the Earth's rotation and the other at right angles to it, each beam would have reached the same distance from the observer after any given lapse of time. With respect to humanity's intuitive understanding of motion and speed, the implications were staggering. They indicated, quite simply, that two observers might be located some distance from one another, both of them falling on a straight line with the front of a propagating light wave. Notwithstanding the separation of the two observers and the linear relation to the light beam, both observers can be equidistant from the wave front. It was difficult for science to absorb the finding, for it suggested something akin to the notion that a thing might be in two places at once.

Einstein's theory of relativity offered an explanation for the findings but required that humanity abandon the Newtonian notion that time was an absolute quantity. Newtonian physics held distance to be a relative matter since two observers might have different velocities. If observer A were moving at one hundred meters per second to the north and observer B were moving at one hundred meters per second southward, they would not agree on how "far away" some third object was located since each would be regarding it from a different frame of reference. In the Newtonian world, time, on the other hand, was independent of reference. Regardless of their positions and velocities, two accurate observers would always agree on the lengths of time intervals. Observer A and B would agree on the length of a second. They would agree on the time at which the sun rose and set regardless of the fact that they might be traveling in opposite directions at different speeds.

Relativity put an end to the concept of absolute time. In the Einsteinian world, two different observers carrying identical clocks could accurately record different times for the occurrence of the same event. Neither would be right and neither would be wrong. A frame of reference carries its own system of time as it does a system of space and distance. The theory of relativity recognizes only one absolute parameter: the speed of light. That is constant in all frames of reference, which constitutes a recognition of the Michelson-Morley findings. Space *and* time are in all other respects relative to perspective.

One of the more vexing implications of Einstein's theory is embodied in the precept that velocity has an absolute limit. Nothing, Einstein concluded, can travel faster than the speed of light. That is not because humanity lacks the resources to construct vehicles capable of such rapid movement (although it does lack such resources), but because the phenomenon of motion has an absolute limit equal to the speed of electromagnetic radiation. In the same way that one cannot have an age less than zero—because there is no such thing—no one and nothing can or ever will be able to travel faster than the speed of light: there is no such thing!

The absolute limit on velocity is tied in with the revolutionary discovery that mass and energy are equivalent. This component of the relativity theory is manifest in the equation $E=mc^2$. It means that all mass is energy, that all energy is mass, and that the two are interconvertible. It means, also, that as an object attains increased speed (by the acquisition of energy), its mass increases as well. At Earthly velocities, the effect is unnoticeable, but if an object were to attain, perhaps, 75 percent of the speed of light, its mass would be appreciably higher than it was at rest. As the object gains increasing amounts of energy and hence approaches the speed of light, its mass approaches infinity and so cannot exceed the speed of light. The infinite mass would require a force of infinite magnitude to produce further acceleration.

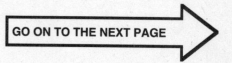
GO ON TO THE NEXT PAGE

32 CRACKING THE MCAT

1. According to the passage, Einstein's theory of relativity states that:

    A. time is absolute for all objects traveling at or near the speed of light.
    B. the speed of light varies, depending on the observer's frame of reference.
    C. time varies for different frames of reference, but the speed of light does not.
    D. time is absolute, but space is not.

2. The author suggests that the theory of relativity:

    A. is inconsistent with Newtonian views of the universe.
    B. contradicts the Michelson-Morley experiment.
    C. is valid only for two observers in the same frame of reference.
    D. cannot be proven right or wrong.

3. The author indicates that under the relativity theory, unlike earlier theories:

    A. mass and energy are conserved only in reactions taking place on Earth.
    B. all mass has the inherent ability to travel faster than light.
    C. neither mass nor energy can ever be converted or destroyed.
    D. energy may be transformed to mass, and mass may be transformed to energy.

4. The fact that most motion we deal with day to day involves speeds far less than that of light means that:

    A. two observers cannot appreciate the fact that their frames of reference may differ.
    B. we are not aware that moving objects experience changes in mass.
    C. we cannot view motion according to the Newtonian model.
    D. we do not perceive any difference between the parameters of space and time.

5. According to the passage, the equation $E = mc^2$ represents:

    A. a new manner of describing a longstanding physical law.
    B. a highly innovative view of the relationship between two well-known parameters.
    C. an alternative formulation of the Michelson-Morley hypothesis.
    D. a direct outgrowth of Newtonian physics.

6. According to Einstein, two observers will agree on the time at which a single event occurs only if:

    A. they are in the same frame of reference.
    B. they apply Newtonian laws of motion.
    C. they refer to clocks of varying mass.
    D. they move in opposite directions at or near the speed of light.

7. Which of the following findings would weaken the theory of relativity as it is described in the passage?

    I. Certain subatomic particles and waves travel at speeds that exceed the speed of light.
    II. The speed of sound is dependent on the medium in which it travels.
    III. No known Earthly object has ever achieved a speed equal to that of light.

    A. I only
    B. III only
    C. I and II only
    D. I, II, and III

GO ON TO THE NEXT PAGE

"Socialization" refers to the processes and dynamics by which children come to understand their position in relation to the positions of others. In the process of socialization, the child learns to respect the rights and
5 property of others. Ideally, he or she recognizes, gradually, the need to control impulses and appetites, to accept and fulfill responsibilities, and to conform behavior to the circumstances that surround him or her at any given time. The six-month-old infant taken by a parent to the theater
10 does not think it inappropriate to cry loudly during the performance, but the six-*year*-old will likely restrain himself even if he is uncomfortable and discontented.

Classical sociologists view the socialization process as occurring in discrete stages. At one stage, it is said, the
15 child learns that he is not the center of all activity and ceases to demand constant attention from adults. Later, he learns to cope with absences and temporary separations. Still further on, he learns something about boundaries and territory—that all things do not belong to him
20 and that his wish is not always another's command. Later still, he comes to appreciate that he is not the only person with unmet needs and later still, develops a bona fide wish to help meet the needs of others. Still further on, the child learns to process complex information at higher levels of
25 reasoning and abstraction.

Matthew Speier, among others perhaps, feels that socialization might be understood in other terms. Specifically, he suggests that the child's integration into his social environment requires, fundamentally, that he learn
30 to *interact*. Speier believes that the achievement of any and all developmental milestones identified by classic sociology (and psychology) reflects a deeper-lying development of *interactional competence*—an ability to conduct communication with the world outside the self.
35 He chose to study socialization in terms of the interactional process and the child's development of an ability to interact.

Speier wrote, "It is my firm belief that no investigation of acquisition processes can effectively get under-
40 way until the concrete features of interactional competencies are analyzed as topics in their own right." He thus sought to reduce human interaction to its essential components in order then to study the child's development of interactional ability. In one of his papers, for example,
45 Speier studied a seemingly simple interaction between an eight-year-old child and his playmate's mother. The child knocked at the front door of the playmate's home. The mother answered and asked who was there. The child did not state his name but instead asked whether "your son"

50 might come out. The mother, in turn, responded that the playmate (her son) was not at home. The child said "O.K." and departed.

With reference to this episode Speier noted that the eight-year-old child had developed some interactional
55 competencies but not others, thus establishing that interactional competence involves the acquisition of discrete skills. The mother had asked the boy to identify himself, but the boy offered no direct response. Instead, he stated his request, which was to have his friend come outside
60 and join him. The child, Speier suggests, had his own purpose in mind and did not fully appreciate the need and propriety of interacting with another in order to pursue it. On the one hand he understood the need to knock at the door and to say something of his purpose to the person
65 who answered, but he did not process the question as to his identity.

Most impressively, however, the child had identified his playmate not by name, but as "your son." That means, first of all, that the child drew conclusions as to the
70 identity of his questioner: He concluded that she was his playmate's mother. Second, he related to this woman in *referent terms* —terms that would refer the interaction to *her*. He did not speak of "Johnny," or "my friend," but to "your son."

75 At the age of eight this child had learned to increase the efficacy of interaction by resorting to references with which the other party is familiar. He had in some primitive fashion coached himself to interact in a way that would be meaningful to the party with whom he sought to
80 communicate. He recognized in some way the need to speak *her* "language." At the same time, however, he had not appreciated the importance of identifying himself in some objective way. Rather, when asked who he was, he simply stated the purpose of his call.

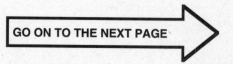
GO ON TO THE NEXT PAGE

8. The author probably compares the situations of a six-month-old and six-year-old taken to the theater in order to demonstrate that:

A. fully socialized adults must take responsibility for less socialized children.
B. children who are exposed to music and art will experience faster maturation.
C. older children have greater appreciation for culture than do younger children.
D. an older child is likely to be more socialized than a younger child.

9. Which of the following statements represents the most sensible use of the information in the passage?

A. Children could begin to study a foreign language at an early age.
B. Schoolteachers could use the information to improve training of reading-disabled children.
C. Parents might use the information to promote more productive interactions among their several children.
D. Sociologists might use the information to expand their understanding of socialization.

10. A social psychologist conducted a study in which one hundred eight-year-olds were observed knocking on a door to call on a playmate. When each child was asked by a parent whom he wished to see, 90 percent identified the playmate by name. Given the discussion in the passage, it is most reasonable to conclude that:

A. some eight-year-olds are far more independent of their parents than others.
B. most eight-year-olds are better able to identify a person by name than by his relationship to others.
C. most eight-year-olds have no concern for the relationship between another child and that child's parent.
D. most eight-year-olds think of themselves as fully independent beings, not as the children of their parents.

11. By the age of six months most children have developed the ability to wave "bye-bye" to departing persons. Professor Speier would most likely view this development as:

A. unrelated to the process of socialization.
B. the achievement of a specific interactional ability.
C. a crucial stage in the child's ability to process information.
D. a reflection of the child's ability to cope with separations and absence.

12. Speier views the situation involving the child who called at his playmate's home (lines 46–53) as demonstrating that:

A. socialization and interaction are entirely separate developmental processes.
B. children are better able to interact with other children than with adults.
C. children do not understand the role they themselves play in interaction.
D. the ability to interact competently with others involves a number of separate interactional abilities.

13. Matthew Speier's views are relevant to sociology because they:

A. suggest a new conceptual framework within which to view the socialization process.
B. name discrete developmental stages by which children can be evaluated.
C. classify all forms of interaction between children and adults.
D. confirm all aspects of the classical view of socialization.

14. The main point of the passage is that:

A. interaction is only one of many competencies that create a fully socialized human being.
B. children of similar age vary sharply in their development because of diverse interactional abilities.
C. it may be possible to understand the socialization process in terms of interactional development.
D. adults should be understanding of children's natural interactional disabilities.

15. As used in the passage, the phrase "referent terms" means:

A. expressions with which people of diverse backgrounds are likely to be familiar.
B. words that enable a listener to relate a subject to himself.
C. phrases that allow a speaker to describe diverse relationships in a single communication.
D. sentences that do not employ proper names.

GO ON TO THE NEXT PAGE

In 1799 William Smith reported that each of the rock formations he had studied featured an individualized group of fossils. Moreover, within each formation, he wrote, "fossils succeed one another in the same order." Smith's observation led geologists to the conclusion that rocks were layered in terms of time, with the deepest-lying layers representing older periods and the superficial representing the more modern. Moreover, the fossils found in a given layer represent life forms of the corresponding period. The modern science of geology depends on the study of the rock strata that Smith identified and the fossils within them.

Rock formations track the history of the Earth and, more particularly, the evolution of life. As earlier, less sophisticated life forms gave rise to later, more sophisticated ones, fossilization within the rocks maintained a record. Indeed, Smith's rock strata are often called, in the aggregate, the "record of the rocks." Geologists describe the record as consisting of six layers. These are the Azoic, Archeozoic, Proterozoic, Paleozoic, Mesozoic, and Cenozoic layers. A corresponding *evolutionary period* was named for each.

The Azoic period is lifeless. Subsequent to the Azoic era life began—in the water. Even much later as life invaded land it continued to evolve and diversify in the sea as it does today. The Archeozoic is a period of single-celled aquatic organisms. Life acquired some greater sophistication during the Proterozoic period, but all Proterozoic life, plant and animal, remained confined entirely to the water. The vast lands of the Proterozoic Earth were absolutely lifeless—as dead and barren in this regard as we imagine to be the surfaces of Pluto, Jupiter, and the moon. A hypothetical visitor to the Proterozoic Earth would doubtless have concluded that life was a phenomenon that was and always would be restricted to water.

In the Paleozoic era life spread into marshy river valleys and along the edges of sea lagoons. Still it remained close to the sea, and the vast masses of land remained lifeless. It was during the Mesozoic period that the record shows great colonization of the land by amphibians and reptiles. Great reptiles (including the dinosaurs) roamed the Earth, and it is undoubted also that small rodentlike mammals were scampering about among the rocks at some distance from the sea during the late (but not early) Mesozoic period. Yet as H. G. Wells wrote, there is no evidence that there existed during the Mesozoic period "any mammal that could look a dinosaur

in the face." Mammals emerged in all their glory during the Cenozoic period, which began some 150 million years ago and continues to the present. The subperiod of their greatest proliferation and predominance is sometimes called "the age of mammals."

The deposition of rock did not occur in truly distinct layers, but as a continuous phenomena. The record of the rocks should appear more as a spectrum of change in which fossils reveal a gradual blending and melding of older life forms into newer ones. Instead the formations do appear as absolutely discrete strata, and the fossils present in any one are sharply different from fossils that appear in those adjacent to it. Undoubtedly the reason for the appearance of discrete rock layers is that the record has been broken at various points because of widespread changes on the Earth that have caused much deposition to be lost to us. Although the record shows us the Cenozoic era as immediate successor to the Mesozoic, there was undoubtedly much that went on between the two periods that is lost to us. The Earth was not one day populated with reptiles and on the next populated with large mammals. The fact that the record should reveal across two layers a near-complete disappearance of an older genus and the appearance of highly evolved organisms of a new and different genus suggests that the entire Earth must have experienced some tremendous cataclysm during which the record was interrupted and most species of the reptile genus were rapidly eliminated–wiped out. The mammalian genus evolved in a world with only a few surviving reptilian species. The *recorded* story of the Cenozoic era begins after the mammals had already achieved a preponderance that must have required an immense amount of time. That unimaginably long period, like those that intervene between the other geologic eras, is lost to our study.

16. Why are geologists unable to study events that occurred between the Mesozoic and Cenozoic era?

   A. The deposition of rock was not a continuous phenomenon.
   B. There was no life during that period.
   C. The rocks provide no record of that interval.
   D. There are no classes intermediate between reptiles and mammals.

GO ON TO THE NEXT PAGE

17. Which of the following is common to Paleozoic and Proterozoic life?

   A. Dependence on proximity to water.
   B. Increased sophistication over Mesozoic organisms.
   C. Presence of small mammals.
   D. Colonization of land masses.

18. The passage suggests that the appearance of rock formations in distinctly identifiable layers means that:

   A. most rock deposits fail to supply meaningful information concerning the evolution of life.
   B. evolution was not as gradual a process as is often believed.
   C. widespread environmental changes prevented some deposits from being preserved.
   D. all life also developed according to discrete stages and periods.

19. Imagine that a newly discovered rock deposit is explored and that geologists are studying fossils contained in the Cenozoic layer. From information contained in the passage, the geologists would be LEAST likely to discover:

   A. prominence of mammalian life forms.
   B. preponderance of great reptilian organisms.
   C. evidence of life expanding beyond bodies of water and shorelines.
   D. a large variety of fish and marine organisms.

20. If an early Paleozoic rock deposit revealed fossils of small mammals, this discovery would weaken which of the following assertions made in the passage?

   I. The age of the mammals was a part of the Cenozoic era.
   II. Mammalian life first appeared in the late Mesozoic era.
   III. Archeozoic life was confined entirely to the water.

   A. I only
   B. II only
   C. I and III only
   D. II and III only

21. According to the passage, the great reptiles were destroyed by a sudden cataclysm with widespread effects across the Earth. On what evidence is this assertion based?

   A. Most mammals living during the Paleozoic period were small.
   B. No reptiles exist on the Earth today.
   C. Some rock deposits present a record of the period between the Mesozoic and Cenozoic in which mammals and reptiles actively competed.
   D. The life forms of the Mesozoic and Cenozoic are dramatically different.

22. If the fossilized remains of an unknown species were found in a Proterozoic rock deposit, one might most reasonably conclude that the organism:

   A. lived in the water.
   B. lived among rock.
   C. had no need for oxygen.
   D. became extinct because of a cataclysmic event.

23. Which of the following observations would best support the hypothesis that reptiles evolved directly from amphibians?

   A. Early amphibians and reptiles differed dramatically from one another in their physiology and behavior.
   B. Fossil remains of the earliest reptiles resemble those of the amphibians.
   C. Most reptiles were extinct before the first amphibians appeared.
   D. Both amphibians and reptiles are represented today by a relatively few species.

24. Among the following, the finding that fossilized whale remains first appear after the great reptiles have disappeared would LEAST support the conclusion that:

   A. whales and reptiles require different environments for their survival.
   B. whales evolved directly from early mammals.
   C. whales evolved from early Cenozoic aquatic animals.
   D. whales and great reptiles co-existed during the Mesozoic era.

GO ON TO THE NEXT PAGE

Federal law will soon require that states articulate guidelines for establishing the size of child support awards to be paid by a noncustodial parent to a custodial parent. The law was enacted in response to a widespread percep-
5 tion that many states lacked meaningful criteria through which child support awards were to be established. In enacting the law, Congress has been generally concerned that child support orders might be either inadequate or unjust. Congress has found that some awards are eco-
10 nomically inadequate to facilitate adequate child rearing. Others reflected a pattern of inconsistency wherein two noncustodial parents similarly situated might find them-selves paying very different child support awards.

As to the matter of inadequacy, a recent study showed
15 that the nation's noncustodial parents would have paid more than $20 billion in 1983 if support awards took realistic account of the cost of child rearing. Census data, however, indicate that only $10.1 billion was due in 1983 and, moreover, that only $7.1 billion was actually paid.
20 The situation thus revealed an *adequacy gap* of $10 billion and a *compliance gap* of $3 billion. Without congressional action, the adequacy gap would likely increase. The compliance gap is likely to increase regard-less.

25 It is a matter of fundamental fairness that like parties should be treated alike. As individuals, most state judges are fairly consistent in the standards and criteria they apply in setting child support awards. Yet studies show that within a given state, judges do not necessarily exhibit
30 similar patterns in setting their awards. The quality of life for a separating couple and their children will depend on the judge who sets the support award rather than on pre-established criteria. It was found that in Colorado one parent might be required to make a support payment
35 equal to 6 percent of income, while a similarly situated parent before another court might be required to pay a full third of income.

As the new federal law takes hold, states face a choice regarding the model on which they wish to base
40 their criteria. The "flat rate" model imposes on all paying parents a payment equal to a flat percentage of income, adjusted for the number of children at issue. Rates might be, for example, 8 percent for one child, 15 percent for two children, and 20 percent for three children. Under
45 such a flat rate structure, all paying parents with one child would pay 8 percent of their income in support. The actual rates, of course, would depend on the states.

Conversely, the "income shares" model embodies the idea that each child should receive that percentage of
50 total parental income as would have been received had the parents not separated. Each parent, in turn, is ex-pected to contribute out of his or her income pro rata according to his or her contribution to total income. Suppose, for example, a separating couple has one child.
55 Spouse A is the custodial spouse and has income of $20,000. Spouse B has income of $60,000, which makes for a total parental income of $80,000. Twenty-five percent of the total derives from spouse A and 75 percent from spouse B. If the court determined that the child
60 would ordinarily enjoy the benefit of 20 percent of total income ($16,000), the parents would be required to provide that amount pro rata. Spouse A would be ex-pected to contribute 25 percent ($4,000), and Spouse B would pay 75 percent ($12,000).

65 Flat rate and income shares awards reflect different values and thus lead to different awards. Where two children live with a payee spouse and the payee spouse has no income, Wisconsin's flat rate approach, for ex-ample, would require monthly payments of $186 from a
70 payor spouse whose monthly income is $600. In the same situation, the income shares approach would require a monthly payment of $90. Because the approach to guide-lines may differ from state to state, guidelines will not bring about parity in support orders across state lines.

25. The passage suggests that the amount of child support that is owed but not paid each year:

   A. will probably increase in spite of congressional action.
   B. is likely to decrease if the adequacy gap is eliminated.
   C. may experience a decrease in response to congressional action.
   D. will remain relatively constant across state lines.

GO ON TO THE NEXT PAGE

26. The author indicates that Congress took action in the area of child support partially in order to:

    A. encourage both custodial and noncustodial parents to assume responsibility for their children's support.

    B. address the fact that noncustodial parents were not complying with support orders.

    C. correct the unfairness produced by state judges who apply diverse criteria in setting awards.

    D. see that all noncustodial parents paid child support in accordance with a single flat rate formula.

27. According to the passage, one aim of the income shares approach to child support is to:

    A. put custodial and noncustodial parents in identical economic positions.

    B. prevent divorce from interfering with the child's economic life.

    C. place the child with the parent best able to provide for him.

    D. ease the economic burden that divorce places on custodial parents.

28. Given the discussion set forth in the passage, one might justifiably conclude that child support awards will:

    A. begin to reflect more objective rather than subjective criteria.

    B. experience a gradual decline as the new federal law operates.

    C. be oriented less toward the needs of the child and more toward the needs of parents.

    D. cease to become an important component of separation and divorce proceedings.

29. Before the new federal law took effect, the passage indicates, a judge's role in setting child support awards might best be described as:

    I. determinative.
    II. relatively insignificant.
    III. largely unregulated.

    A. I only
    B. II only
    C. I and III only
    D. I, II, and III

30. The passage indicates that similarly situated parents in different states may continue to experience different treatment because:

    I. judges are unlikely to abandon their own personal opinions in favor of legal criteria.

    II. separate states may adopt divergent criteria for setting support awards.

    III. the flat rate model does not take account of the custodial parent's income.

    A. I only
    B. II only
    C. I and III only
    D. I, II, and III

GO ON TO THE NEXT PAGE

Frequently we refer to "commitment" without appreciating its meaning or its significance to individuals and the social structure as a whole. What is the role of commitment in human life? Indeed, what *is* commit-
5 ment? It is probably not correct to think of commitment as one among many valuable character traits. Rather, commitment is the fundamental underpinning of all valuable character traits. In the absence of commitment, human existence would represent no more than vegeta-
10 tive life.

The *development of charact*er fully depends on commitment. In order to gain an identity—a true self—a person must make choices day to day, month to month, and year to year. Many of these choices have irreversible
15 consequences and so commit the individual to one course or another. The need to make such choices may produce pleasure, or it may produce anguish. But such is the fabric of character. In terms of moral structure one is, in fact, the product of his or her decisions. Therein does humanity
20 differ from other forms of life. The kernel becomes a corn plant simply on the basis of programmed genetic development: The plant makes no decisions. The puppy gives rise to the dog through aging and physical growth, not through will. Only men and women attain their selfhood
25 by virtue of decision making, and decision making imports commitment. Arnold Howe describes commitment as the sine qua non of social life. It makes us what we are.

Commitment takes a variety of forms. When most people consider commitment, they probably think of one
30 who gives time and energy to a particular activity. This is certainly a type of commitment. One may devote herself to a social cause, to the welfare of some other person or persons, to her own professional endeavors, or, perhaps, to a hobby. There is also, however, a creature
35 called "societal commitment." Persons with societal commitment generally promote values of tolerance and pluralism. They reject violence and they persevere in the face of antagonism and adversity. Seralius, for example, continued to write his essays despite imprisonment and
40 torture. Those with societal commitment seem to possess a genuine ability to feel for others. Often that ability is a product of the suffering they themselves have endured.

There is also a thing that might be called interpersonal commitment. One makes this kind of commitment
45 when one allows oneself truly to trust another person. Sometimes the trust leads to intimacy and sometimes to enmity. One can never know in advance how another person might use or abuse one's trust. The only certainty
is that having trusted another, one will not remain un-
50 changed. Hence, trust constitutes taking an irreversible course of action, the consequences of which are not known a priori. Interpersonal commitment differs from societal commitment. The latter involves the quest for a better civilization. The former involves the investment of
55 one's self in another.

Commitment is not only the basis of character, it is a prerequisite to art, literature, music, and even to technological and economic progress. No socially useful product or advance is achieved without a commitment on
60 some person's behalf. The writer chooses to write and thus forgoes other professional pursuits. The scientific researcher, the entrepreneur, and the financier likewise make decisions to direct their inspiration to some particular pursuit, and those decisions ultimately create insight
65 and innovation.

31. According to the passage, commitment is a quality that:

A. means more to an individual than to a society.
B. is the root of animal and vegetable life.
C. is a substructure, not a trait.
D. has no fundamental underpinnings.

32. The author states that interpersonal commitment is distinct from societal commitment. From the information in the passage, this statement is probably based on the author's belief that:

A. interpersonal commitment requires that one person put faith in another.
B. interpersonal commitment usually leads to intimacy.
C. societal commitment requires no genuine concern for others.
D. societal commitment requires no investment.

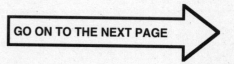
GO ON TO THE NEXT PAGE

33. To illustrate a difference between humans and other living things, the author describes the "development of character" (line 11). He wishes to indicate that:

    A. selfhood is attained through commitment to social good.

    B. plants, although living, cannot be said to make commitments.

    C. commitment is essential to the human identity.

    D. human beings are fated to be social beings regardless of their own decisions.

34. As described in the passage, Arnold Howe's description of commitment as the sine qua non of social life most probably indicates that:

    A. indecision is the cause of most human misery.

    B. emotional growth and development are furthered by decision making and commitment.

    C. selfhood is attained through devotion to social causes.

    D. only humans are capable of programmed genetic development.

35. Based on the passage, which of the following would most WEAKEN the claim that only humans must make commitments in order to develop their characters?

    A. Proof that dogs can reason abstractly.

    B. Evidence that animals experience lasting gratification and pain over the need to make choices.

    C. Indications that all animals have certain inborn instincts.

    D. Documentation that the frontal lobes of some animals are more intricately convoluted than human frontal lobes.

36. It is said that commitment requires persistence. What assertion does the passage make in support of such an idea?

    A. All hobbies require skill that takes years to develop.

    B. People are required to make choices in life.

    C. Seralius continued to write even though he was tortured.

    D. There can be no commitment of energy without a commitment of time.

37. The ability to empathize, according to the passage, is most closely identified with:

    A. increasing openness.

    B. societal commitment.

    C. meaningful intimacy.

    D. the possession of hope.

GO ON TO THE NEXT PAGE

In the absence of government there is chaos. This fact endows government with its essential purpose: the creation and maintenance of order. The price of order is liberty, and the various forms of government that history
5 has seen differ in the compromises they strike between these two competing interests. The varied forms of human government (dictatorship, and democracy, for example) differ considerably in the way they treat the contest between order and liberty. They differ also in the
10 degrees of benefit and harm they visit on their peoples.

An oligarchy is a government wherein power is vested in a chosen minority. The "choosing" might be done on the basis of birth, in which case the oligarchy is termed an aristocracy. It might, on the other hand, be
15 based on religious affiliation, in which case we call the government a theocracy. The word "democracy," with its root "*demos,*" implies that "power is vested in the people." Yet in most functioning democracies the wealthy tend to hold public office, and it is perhaps correct to consider
20 modern democracies as a species of oligarchy.

Of all forms of government, democracy demands the most of its people. It requires, above all, competent voting mentalities—a voting population with sufficient insight and understanding to understand where its own
25 best interests lie. Left to his own devices, a small child is likely to prefer a caretaker who proclaims that an undisciplined life of play, frolic, and indulgence will lead to happiness. He will disbelieve those who seek to impose sensible limits and discipline. Similarly, when voters are
30 uneducated, misinformed, and unthinking, they might distrust a well-meaning and competent government and be duped by an evil one. Attempts to foster democratic governments in underdeveloped nations where the great majority of people are illiterate invariably fail, and despo-
35 tism in one way or another takes over. One cynic remarked that "you mustn't enthrone ignorance just because there is so much of it."

Yet where democracy does succeed, it is clearly the most promising form of government. The historical
40 record is plain on this point. Modern Western democracies are responsible for most of the progress that the world now enjoys. It is in the democracies, not the monarchies or other forms of dictatorship, that science and the arts have best flourished. In the ancient world, Athens and
45 Rome set similar examples. Their governments promoted the most productive and innovative societies that history had then known.

Moreover, it seems that successful democracy is stronger than any other form of government. In recent
50 history, at any rate, democratic powers have tended to previl in armed conflicts (such as WWII), and are, furthermore often the prime movers for peace. People who more or less control their own destinies *want* peace. Others, it seems, may not, or they may be more easily
55 talked into war.

In order to promote democracy throughout the world, today's living democracies must strive to educate the world's peoples. Most people truly interested in spreading democracy recognize that food, clothing, and shelter
60 are prerequisites to education. For peoples who lack these basic necessities, the world's free societies should band together and try to provide them. Their goal, however, should be to provide basic necessities in order then to provide schooling, for an educated world is the
65 only sort that will be seriously receptive to democratic ideals.

Here in the United States it remains to be seen whether democracy can survive in the face of grossly unequal wealth distribution. Domestic poverty has in the
70 past produced urban riots and violent protest. The American government has generally responded with social programs designed to address the problem. Yet a cycle of violent protest and governmental action is of dubious viability. Notwithstanding its awesome military power,
75 one might wonder whether the present form of government can endure in the absence of some meaningful and permanent change in the disparate economic status of diverse portions of the population.

38. The example concerning the small child (lines 25–29) is designed to demonstrate that:

A. education is more important than freedom.
B. where people have a meaningful choice between candidates, democracy will succeed.
C. uninformed voters are easily misled.
D. education is more easily made equal in a disciplined society.

GO ON TO THE NEXT PAGE

39. Based on the passage, the government that has the best chance of surviving is:

- A. an oligarchy ruled by a minority.
- B. a democracy whose citizens are well educated.
- C. a well-intentioned monarchy.
- D. a dictatorship.

40. The author refers to attempts to foster democracies in underdeveloped nations in order, primarily, to make the point that:

- A. no one can govern effectively without understanding the needs of the people.
- B. democracy cannot succeed without a well-informed population.
- C. education is the most important of all human values.
- D. in all forms of government there are those who would seek to gain power by deception.

41. Based on the passage, the view that a democracy vests power "in the people" (lines 16–17) is:

- A. widely disbelieved.
- B. thoroughly unsupported by historical evidence.
- C. a deception that the wealthy perpetrate on the poor.
- D. probably unjustified.

42. According to the passage, most people who wish to spread democracy probably would NOT agree that:

- A. education can flourish in the face of poverty.
- B. learning depends on physical well-being.
- C. poverty must be addressed before learning can proceed.
- D. education is a prerequisite to political freedom.

43. The cynic who remarked that "ignorance [must not be] enthroned" (lines 35–37) probably meant that:

- A. in a monarchy ignorance has a way of perpetuating itself.
- B. ignorant politicians will harm their nations even if they are well meaning.
- C. majority rule can be disadvantageous to a public that is not well educated.
- D. in a true democracy all people should be entitled to vote regardless of education.

44. Based on information in the passage, one reason that the American government might ultimately deteriorate is that it:

- A. is overly concerned with military strength and inadequately concerned with individual rights.
- B. strives to offer too much to too many.
- C. has not solved the problem of economic inequality.
- D. has not dealt appropriately with violence.

GO ON TO THE NEXT PAGE

Prior to the onset of industrial capitalism material neediness was the rule. People simply did not own very much. Possessions that would be considered quite commonplace today were scarce. Cookware, utensils, tablecloths, and such were privileges of the wealthy. The commoner owned very few such articles. William Shakespeare wrote in his will that his "second-best bed" should go to Anne Hathaway. Such, apparently, was one of the prized possessions of the world's greatest writer.

The essence of capitalism is in the fact that it seeks out unmet economic needs and undertakes to meet them. Capitalism is not concerned with class. It is concerned with sales. That explains how capitalism facilitated the industrial revolution of the nineteenth century. Material possessions were in demand, but there was little supply. Simple dynamics of the market made it possible for anyone to grow rich if he could produce at an affordable price an abundance of relatively simple household articles. Such people were the early industrial capitalists who fomented the industrial revolution. Widespread material neediness gave them the incentive to direct technological know-how toward the production of goods in demand.

With the onslaught of the industrial revolution, *things* began to flow from factories to the society at large. People began to enjoy an ever-widening variety of products to which they were not accustomed. Clothing, paper, furniture, pens, curtains, and the like became available not just to the wealthy, but also to the middle class and even to the poor. This in turn gave rise to what we would call a broad-based increase in the standard of living.

Concomitant with the flood of consumer goods were ongoing improvements to the industrial apparatus. Instruments of production became increasingly more efficient and sophisticated. Consider the iron industry. In the 1770s the usual furnace designed to extract ore was ten feet high. By 1870 it was ten times that height. Similarly, the crucibles designed for the production of steel experienced precipitous growth. At the end of the eighteenth century the typical crucible was as large as a water bottle. One hundred years later it was as large as a dwelling. Individual looms were transformed into gargantuan mills. Mass output was the order of the day.

The industrial revolution ushered in the era of automation and divided labor, and thus altered, forever, the nature of employment. Before the industrial era a single artisan might have made an entire product unassisted and without the use of sophisticated machinery. The furniture maker made the entire cabinet, and he did so by hand. The carriage maker made the whole carriage with only the tools he could hold in his ten fingers. As production en masse took hold, such use of labor was shown to be inefficient. Specialization was the trend, and machinery became important. The production of a carriage required one person who made nothing but wheels, another who made nothing but chassis, another who made seats, and another who made carriage tops. No one person would produce the whole product. People produced pieces of products and other people assembled the pieces. Technology allowed many men and women to realize their aspirations for material wealth, but it also invested their work with monotony.

45. It may be sensibly inferred from the passage that early industrial capitalists would have regarded the scarcity of material wealth that surrounded them as:

    A. positive, because it maintained the class structure to which they were accustomed.
    B. positive, because it provided a ready and lucrative market for their products.
    C. negative, because it signified an abundance of unmet economic needs.
    D. negative, because it diminished opportunities for industrial expansion.

46. One may assume from information in the passage that capitalists profited from improved technology because they were:

    A. shrewd in their ability to create demand for the goods they produced.
    B. able to increase the availability of goods that were wanted.
    C. self-sufficient and hard-working individuals.
    D. aware of the need to ameliorate the plight of the poor.

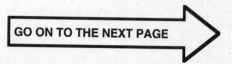
GO ON TO THE NEXT PAGE

47. A reasonable inference from the passage would be that technological advances are attributable in part to:

   A. an increased standard of living.
   B. market forces.
   C. political revolutions based on economic need.
   D. freeing individuals from the necessity of performing repetitive work.

48. Implied in the passage is the assumption that advancing technology contributed to:

   A. a decreased standard of living for the worker.
   B. a longer work day.
   C. increased prevalence of consumer services as opposed to consumer goods.
   D. loss of the artisan's ability to create, on his own, a complete product.

49. The passage asserts that the industrial revolution achieved:

   A. better relations between rich and poor.
   B. an improved standard of living.
   C. increased worker creativity.
   D. greater regard for the value of prosperity.

50. The passage states that the industrial revolution produced specialization and automation. It is reasonable to assume that these trends caused:

   I. some people to realize their dreams.
   II. some very large manufacturing companies to become obsolete.
   III. some laborers to work in a way to which they were not accustomed.

   A. I only
   B. II only
   C. I and II only
   D. I and III only

51. The passage asserts that furnaces for extracting iron ore greatly increased in size. It is reasonable to conclude that this probably contributed to:

   A. decreased use of wood and steel.
   B. increased use and production of iron.
   C. an overall decrease in industrial wages.
   D. a sharp increase in the employment rate.

GO ON TO THE NEXT PAGE

African art includes houses, masks, costumes, uniforms, and the decorations that adorn clothing. We cannot understand it without first abandoning some conventional notions. African art goes beyond monuments and beyond that which one might observe in a museum.

The mbari house is filled with sculptures and probably represents a religious offering. The construction of the house is conducted in ritualistic fashion, and, once built, the house and its sculptures are never maintained. They are permitted to deteriorate and to become once again a part of the ground from which they came. Typically, a mbari house contains upwards of seventy sculptures. Usually the sculptures depict significant deities of the community. The front of a mbari house, for example, will usually feature the sculpted figure of the goddess of the Earth. The sculpture is a veritable complex showing not only the goddess herself, but also her children seated nearby. Her servants, too, are figured in poses that clearly illustrate their function as her guards. Away from the front of the house other sculptures are usually found. These may assume a variety of forms. They may represent gods and they may depict human figures of myth or history.

Close to the Ivory Coast, there lives a tribe called "Dan." The Dan are inveterate mask makers and have what amounts to a mask-making club that they call "poro." Masks play a significant role in the operation of Dan society. Members of poro tend to hold functional political offices, and they generally regulate community affairs. They wear masks while executing their functions, and community regard for the masks aids them in their work as does the anonymity that the mask provides. For example, the Dan have developed a mask that represents justice or judging, and the community judge, a member of poro, wears the mask when performing his official function. Other functionaries called on to perform unpopular tasks are similarly protected by anonymity when they wear the masks that represent their offices.

The Yoruba *Gelade* is another mask-making group. *Gelade* refers to a mysterious group of persons who devote themselves to the appeasement of gods whom they believe to be the sponsors of witchcraft. *Gelade* masks are costumes and nothing more. They are worn by masqueraders who don them in connection with performances and cult activities. The masks themselves represent a diverse number of personages with whom the Yoruba are familiar. Some masks represent merchants. Others represent motorists, hunters, physicians, and in general, the varied array of characters to whom the Yoruba are exposed. The *Gelade* give performances in which they use the masks to partake of social commentary. In this respect, then, the masks constitute graphic art, and the performances constitute literature.

One should not try to understand African art by resorting to the usual classifications and subdivisions. The classifications "fine art," "decorative art," and "craft" do not do it justice. The African culture differs from the European in that artwork is not separate from utilitarian objects. The designation "African art" describes elaborately adorned eating utensils, simple furniture, clothing, usable pottery, and basketry. African art is thus an "art of life."

52. The information in the passage is organized according to the:

    A. communal participation in art forms.
    B. enduring quality and value of African art.
    C. varied forms of African art.
    D. influence of geographical region on art form.

53. On the basis of statements made in the passage, one is justified in concluding that the mbari house is largely built to:

    A. honor the gods.
    B. celebrate the Earth.
    C. preserve history.
    D. endure as a religious monument.

54. Based on the passage, it is reasonable to conclude that the masks of the Dan tribe differ from those of the Yoruba *Gelade* in that a Dan mask:

    A. might accurately describe the role of the person who wears it.
    B. is never designed by the person who wears it.
    C. has little relationship to social function.
    D. is more bewildering in its form.

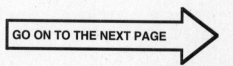
GO ON TO THE NEXT PAGE

55. Based on the passage, which of the following would likely characterize the mbari house?

    I. sparse distribution of religiously oriented sculptures.
   II. representations of deities and associated figures.
  III. wear and disrepair.

    A. I only
    B. II only
    C. III only
    D. II and III only

56. In referring to African art as an "art of life" (paragraph 5), the author probably means that African works of art:

    A. are rigorously classified by African artists.
    B. include articles used in the course of daily life.
    C. are primarily religious in nature.
    D. are not valued by the general African public.

57. It can be reasonably concluded from the passage that the poro are able to manage community affairs largely because their masks:

    I. command great respect from the tribespeople.
   II. shield their identities.
  III. have little relationship to their function.

    A. I only
    B. II only
    C. I and II only
    D. I, II, and III

58. The fact that some art critics insist that all art must be divorced from utilitarian function would most directly challenge the assumption that:

    A. African sculpture has religious significance.
    B. African eating implements constitute art.
    C. Yoruba masks have social significance.
    D. art is best held in collections or museums.

GO ON TO THE NEXT PAGE

How do I explain Zen to a Westerner? It is difficult. Perhaps this is because it is the antithesis of modern Western values. Western culture values ambition, productivity, competition, and acquisition. It values youth over age, and mortality is its enemy. To exaggerate a little, perhaps, Westerners wish their lives to be filled with conquest and to last forever. Anxiety, conflict, and combat are often the consequences. Zen puts a premium on peace, humility, and understanding. It values devotion to work and to creation, but it does not pretend that anyone or anything is permanent. It promotes neither ritual nor formalism. Meditation, which it encourages, is not a ceremony but a purposeful activity. One meditates in order to understand oneself.

A lifelong follower who had studied with several masters once described Zen as "a special teaching without scriptures, beyond words and letters, pointing to the mind-essence of the human being, seeing directly into one's nature, attaining enlightenment. . . ." "Continued involvement in daily events and appreciation of minute occurrences," he submitted, "are elements of 'the way.'" Hence, Zen means many things, none of them fully describable except by the experience itself.

Unquestionably, that which Zen seeks to achieve for the follower is of great worth, and Westerners might do well to explore it. Zen, it is said, brings an end to fear, doubt, and disappointment. The man who honestly views his own passing as the simple falling of a leaf in autumn has very little to fear; who does not seek to outshine or outdo others has little cause for disappointment; who understands himself has nothing to doubt.

All that glitters is not gold, however, and all that is called "Zen" is not necessarily the genuine article. There are societies that have latched on to the word "Zen" without adopting its philosophical framework. Indeed, to some extent Zen has acquired a reputation for the same formalism and fetishism that tends to characterize Western religious practice. In China and Japan, Zen represents itself through ornate temples, priests, monks, wealth, and prestige. Its trappings are the very things it is designed to transcend.

Perhaps I can best describe the essence of Zen by relating a famed Zen story:

There was a Zen master named Hakuin, and he was known by his community as one who lived a pure life. There was in the neighborhood a beautiful young girl who worked in a food store owned by her parents. The girl's parents discovered one day that she was with child. They became angry and demanded to know who was the father. After great hesitancy the daughter named Hakuin, the Zen master.

The girl's parents went to confront Hakuin. They told him that their daughter had named him as the father of her unborn child. Hakuin made no assertion regarding the matter and said only this: "Is that so?" When the child was born, the parents brought it to Hakuin demanding that he care for it. Hakuin had by this time fallen to some disgrace on account of the episode. This did not concern him, and he devoted himself to taking care of the child. From various neighbors he managed to acquire milk and other things the child needed.

About a year later the girl revealed to her parents that the father of the child was not Hakuin but a boy who worked in the store. The parents returned to Hakuin to make their apology and to take the baby back. They explained that the daughter had told them that Hakuin was not the father. As Hakuin yielded the baby he said only, "Is that so?" Preferring not to face Hakuin any longer, the parents departed.

59. The writer of the passage seems to believe that Western values:

   A. contribute to tension and hostility among people.
   B. are competitive with Zen values.
   C. produce only unhappiness.
   D. are the product of anxiety and conflict.

60. The general point made by the author's comparison of Zen with Western culture is that:

   A. Westerners should incorporate Zen into all facets of their daily lives.
   B. Zen promotes a more natural and tranquil existence than does western culture.
   C. the drive to succeed usually produces tension and hostility.
   D. Western values are more easily understood than Zen values.

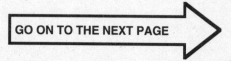
GO ON TO THE NEXT PAGE

61. According to the author, Western culture regards mortality as its enemy. The word "enemy" in this context implies that:

    I. Western culture is constantly preoccupied with battle.

    II. Westerners do not accept death as a natural part of life.

    III. Westerners wish to prolong their youth and their lives.

    A. I only
    B. III only
    C. I and II only
    D. II and III only

62. The fact that Hakuin says only, "Is that so," both times he meets the girl's parents is significant because it shows that he:

    I. rejects what the parents are saying to him.

    II. is not concerned with proving himself right or proving others wrong.

    III. is willing to ask questions but never to make assertions.

    A. I only
    B. II only
    C. III only
    D. I, II, and III

63. The passage indicates that a person who does not compete with others probably will:

    A. be satisfied with what he is and what he has.
    B. embrace Western and Zen philosophies alike.
    C. be suspicious of that which appears to have value.
    D. care for others more than he cares for himself.

64. The passage indicates that on hearing Hakuin's last statement to them, the father and mother most likely experienced

    I. embarrassment and remorse.

    II. bewilderment.

    III. resentment.

    A. I only
    B. II only
    C. III only
    D. II and III only

65. The author appears to blame the fact that Zen has achieved some reputation for formalism on:

    I. the way in which Zen is represented in China and Japan.

    II. people who claim to follow Zen but do not truly embrace it.

    III. the overbearing character of Western culture.

    A. I only
    B. II only
    C. I and II only
    D. I, II, and III

STOP
IF YOU FINISH BEFORE TIME IS CALLED, YOU MAY CHECK YOUR WORK ON THIS TEST ONLY.
DO NOT TURN TO ANY OTHER TEST IN THIS BOOK.

Physical Sciences

Time: 100 Minutes
Questions 1–77

PHYSICAL SCIENCES

DIRECTIONS: Most questions in the Physical Sciences test are organized into groups, each preceded by a descriptive passage. After studying the passage, select the one best answer to each question in the group. Some questions are not based on a descriptive passage and are also independent of each other. You must also select the one best answer to these questions. If you are not certain of an answer, eliminate the alternatives that you know to be incorrect and then select an answer from the remaining alternatives. Indicate your selection by blackening the corresponding circle on your answer sheet (DIAGNOSTIC TEST FORM). A periodic table is provided for your use. You may consult it whenever you wish.

PERIODIC TABLE OF THE ELEMENTS

1 **H** 1.0																	2 **He** 4.0
3 **Li** 6.9	4 **Be** 9.0											5 **B** 10.8	6 **C** 12	2 **N** 14.0	8 **O** 16	9 **F** 19.0	10 **Ne** 20.0
11 **Na** 22.0	12 **Mg** 24.3											13 **Al** 27.0	14 **Si** 28.1	15 **P** 31.0	16 **S** 32.1	17 **Cl** 35.5	18 **Ar** 39.0
19 **K** 39.1	20 **Ca** 40.1	21 **Sc** 45.0	22 **Ti** 47.9	23 **V** 50.9	24 **Cr** 52.0	25 **Mn** 54.9	26 **Fe** 55.8	27 **Co** 58.9	28 **Ni** 58.7	29 **Cu** 63.5	30 **Zn** 65.4	31 **Ga** 69.7	32 **Ge** 72.6	33 **As** 74.9	34 **Se** 79.0	35 **Br** 79.9	36 **Kr** 83.8
37 **Rb** 85.5	38 **Sr** 87.6	39 **Y** 88.9	40 **Zr** 91.2	41 **Nb** 92.9	42 **Mo** 95.9	43 **Tc** 97.0	44 **Ru** 101.0	45 **Rh** 102.9	46 **Pd** 106.4	47 **Ag** 107.9	48 **Cd** 112.4	49 **In** 114.8	50 **Sn** 118.7	51 **Sb** 121.8	52 **Te** 127.6	53 **I** 126.9	54 **Xe** 131.3
55 **Cs** 132.9	56 **Ba** 137.3	57 **La** 138.9	72 **Hf** 178.5	73 **Ta** 180.9	74 **W** 183.9	75 **Re** 186.2	76 **Os** 190.2	77 **Ir** 192.2	78 **Pt** 195.1	79 **Au** 197.0	80 **Hg** 200.6	81 **Tl** 204.4	82 **Pb** 207.2	83 **Bi** 209.0	84 **Po** 209.0	85 **At** 210.0	86 **Rn** 222.0
87 **Fr** 223.0	88 **Ra** 226.0	89 **Ac** 227.0															

58 **Ce** 140.1	59 **Pr** 140.9	60 **Nd** 144.2	61 **Pm** 145.0	62 **Sm** 150.4	63 **Eu** 152.0	64 **Gd** 157.3	65 **Tb** 158.9	66 **Dy** 162.5	67 **Ho** 164.9	68 **Er** 167.3	69 **Tm** 168.9	70 **Yb** 173.0	71 **Lu** 175.0
90 **Th** 232.0	91 **Pa** 231.0	92 **U** 238.0	93 **Np** 237.0	94 **Pu** 244.0	95 **Am** 243.0	96 **Cm** 247.0	97 **Bk** 247.0	98 **Cf** 251.0	99 **Es** 254.0	100 **Fm** 253.0	101 **Md** 256.0	102 **No** 253.0	103 **Lr** 257.0

Acid rain is the accumulation of a high concentration of acids in the atmosphere that results from the interaction of nitrogen and sulfur oxides to produce acids. The emission of sulfur dioxide and nitrogen oxide from power plants combine with other compounds to form complex chemical reactions. The reaction rate is most rapid in the liquid phase. Sulfur dioxide can be converted to sulfur trioxide when it combines with reactive substances such as ozone when solar radiation is absorbed.

The chemistry of acid rain is shown below:

$$SO_3 + H_2O \rightarrow H_2SO_4$$

Reaction I

SO_3 is extremely reactive and, in the presence of water, produces H_2SO_4. This reaction leads to the liberation of heat. Liquid H_2SO_4 boils at 290° C.

Gaseous H_2SO_4 dissociates into SO_3 and water vapor at about 350°C and a pressure of 300 atm.

Sulfuric acid is an extremely important chemical product. It can act as a strong oxidizing agent when it reacts with metals.

$$H_2SO_4 + Ag \rightarrow Ag_2SO_4 + SO_2 + H_2O$$

Reaction II

At high boiling points it can also react with salts to liberate volatile acids such as HCl.

$$H_2SO_4 + NaCl \rightarrow HCl + NaHSO_4$$

Reaction III

1. The balanced equation of Reaction II should be:

   A. $2H_2SO_4 + 4Ag \rightarrow 2Ag_2SO_4 + SO_2 + H_2O.$
   B. $2H_2SO_4 + 2Ag \rightarrow Ag_2SO_4 + SO_2 + 2H_2O.$
   C. $3H_2SO_4 + 2Ag \rightarrow Ag_2SO_4 + 2\ SO_2 + 3H_2O.$
   D. $H_2SO_4 + Ag \rightarrow \frac{1}{2}Ag_2SO_4 + \frac{1}{2}SO_2 + 2H_2O.$

2. Which one of the following is a Lewis base?

   A. HSO_4^-
   B. SO_2
   C. SO_3
   D. H_3O^+

3. A solution of which two species will most resist a change in the pH when a strong base is added to it?

   A. $Ag_2SO_4 : SO_2$
   B. $H_2SO_4 : SO_3$
   C. $H_2SO_4 : NaHSO_4$
   D. $AgCl : NaCl$

4. By definition, a Bronsted-Lowry acid is:

   A. any substance capable of acting as a proton acceptor.
   B. any electron-pair acceptor.
   C. any electron-pair donor.
   D. any substance capable of acting as a source of protons.

5. Sodium chloride has a higher bond dissociation energy than HCl or H_2O because:

   A. NaCl is of a higher molecular weight than HCl or H_2O.
   B. NaCl is covalently bonded and does not have as great a dipole movement as HCl or H_2O have.
   C. NaCl is not a proton donor like HCl or H_2O.
   D. the electrostatic attractive forces are greater between the ions of NaCl than forces within HCl or H_2O.

GO ON TO THE NEXT PAGE

6. An aqueous solution of H_2SO_4 is titrated with a 0.1 M solution of sodium hydroxide, as shown below. Which of the following is true at point 2?

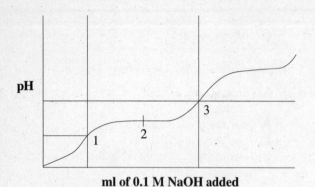

ml of 0.1 M NaOH added

   A.   The concentration of HSO_4^- equals that of SO_4^{-2}.
   B.   The major species in solution are Na^+ and HSO_4^-.
   C.   The pH is equal to the acid dissociation constant of H_2SO_4.
   D.   Point 2 is the first equivalence point.

7. At a temperature of 350° C and a pressure of 320 atm, a sample of 1 mole of H_2SO_4 has completely dissociated into gaseous SO_3 and H_2O. Approximately what is the ratio of the velocities of these two molecules? (M.W. of SO_3 is 80 g/mol.)

   A. $2\sqrt{3}$
   B. $\dfrac{3\sqrt{2}}{2}$
   C. $1\sqrt{5}$
   D. $\dfrac{3\sqrt{5}}{10}$

8. Assuming Reaction I is at equilibrium, which of the following changes will cause an increase in the concentration of sulfuric acid?

   A.   Decreasing the pressure
   B.   Decreasing the concentration of SO_3
   C.   The addition of a catalyst
   D.   Decreasing the temperature

Passage II (Questions 9–16)

   A magnetic field can be used to identify many types of charged particles. In the following experiment, particles were sent into a magnetic field perpendicular to the field's direction and perpendicular to the force of gravity. The figure below shows the forces on a negatively charged particle, P, of charge q and mass m as it first enters the magnetic field along path Y.

   The magnetic field is directed into the page, which is signified by the symbol $\otimes$ for vector B.

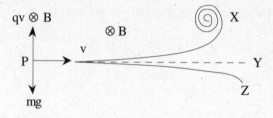

   All charged particles experience a force when moving through a magnetic field. The direction of the force can be found by using the right-hand rule and crossing the particle's direction of motion and the direction of the magnetic field. The magnitude of this force is given by the following equation:

$$F = Bqv \sin q$$

   The angle θ is the angle between the direction of the particle's velocity and the direction of the magnetic field.

   When a relatively low energy particle is sent into the magnetic field it is observed to travel a spiral path that degenerates in a circular fashion as shown for particle X in the figure above. The circular nature of the motion is attributable to the fact that the predominant force experienced by the particle is always perpendicular to the direction of the motion.

   In this experiment two particles are fired into the magnetic field in the direction of path Y. Particle X spirals upward, and particle Z is deflected downward.

   Assume the acceleration due to gravity is 9.8 m/s².

GO ON TO THE NEXT PAGE

9. A particle is fired into the magnetic field. Its initial velocity has components along path Y and into the page. The angle the particle's velocity vector makes with path Y is called phi. Phi can assume values between 0 and $\frac{\pi}{2}$. Which of the following graphs best represents the dependence of the magnitude of the force on the particle to angle phi?

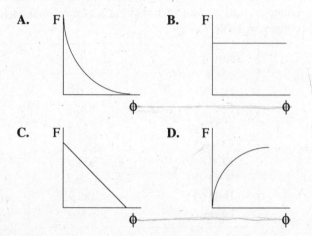

A.

B.

C.

D.

10. Keeping all other factors constant, what changes could be made so particle X traveled in a larger spiral?

    A. Increase the density of the magnetic field.
    B. Give the particle more kinetic energy.
    C. Give the particle less kinetic energy.
    D. Increase the charge on the particle.

11. Particle Z is given an initial velocity of 1×10^3 m/s along path Y. If the field density is 5.5 T and particle Z has a charge of 1 coul, how strong will the net force on the particle be when it first enters the field?

    A. 0 N
    B. 5.5×10^3 N
    C. 1.1×10^3 N
    D. 2.5×10^3 N

12. Particle X spirals inward instead of revolving around a fixed point because:

    A. the particle's velocity is increasing.
    B. the particle is losing energy.
    C. the particle is negatively charged.
    D. the net force on the particle is perpendicular to the plane formed by its velocity vector and the direction of the magnetic field.

13. If particle P were also given a velocity component into the page equal to the magnitude of its velocity in the direction of path Y, the force first felt by the particle would:

    A. decrease by a factor of $\frac{2}{\sqrt{2}}$.

    B. decrease by a factor of $\frac{1}{\sqrt{2}}$.

    C. remain the same.

    D. increase by a factor of $\sqrt{2}$.

14. Assume the magnetic field density is 5.5 T. A large charged object of mass 1 kg and charge 1 coul is sent into the magnetic field along path Y. How fast would the object have to be traveling so the force of the magnetic field and the force of gravity were in equilibrium?

    A. 0.6 m/s
    B. 1.8 m/s
    C. 5.4 m/s
    D. 2.7 m/s

GO ON TO THE NEXT PAGE

15. A particle of mass .001 kg and charge 1 coul enters the magnetic field traveling 1000 m/s. The particle spirals and comes to a complete stop relative to the field in 0.05 s. Neglecting the force of gravity, this event represents work equal to:

    A.   20 J.
    B.   25 J.
    C.   500 J.
    D.   10000 J.

16. The following diagrams represent the path of a negative test-charge moving from point A to point B inside the electric field produced by a negatively charged particle. Which path requires the most amount of work to move the test charge?

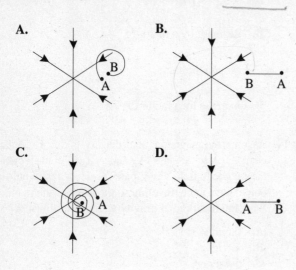

A.

B.

C.

D.

Passage III (Questions 17–23)

A chemist conducted experiments to determine the heat of formation and the Gibbs' free energy for eight substances: H_2, Fe_2O_3, C_2H_4, CO_2, $KClO_4$, N_2O_4, H_2O, and Fe.

Experiment 1

Each substance was synthesized from its constituent elements, and its heat of formation was measured and recorded in Table 1.

Substance	H_f° (kJ/mol)
H_2 (g)	0.0
Fe_2O_3 (c)	−824.2
C_2H_4 (g)	52.3
CO_2 (g)	−393.5
$KClO_4$ (c)	−432.8
N_2O_4 (g)	9.2
H_2O (l)	−285.9
Fe (s)	0.0

(c) = crystalline; (g) = gaseous; (s) = solid; (l) = liquid

Table 1

Experiment 2

For each synthesis studied in Experiment 1, the change in entropy was measured and the Gibbs' free energy was calculated. The results are tabulated in Table 2.

Substance	G_f° (kJ/mol)
H_2 (g)	0.0
Fe_2O_3 (c)	−742.2
C_2H_4 (g)	68.2
CO_2 (g)	−394.4
$KClO_4$ (c)	−303.1
N_2O_4 (g)	97.9
H_2O (l)	−236.8
Fe (s)	0.0

Table 2

GO ON TO THE NEXT PAGE

17. Which of the following events in a synthesis reaction describes a decrease in entropy?

   A.. The number of moles of product is more than the number of moles of reactants.
   B. The number of moles of product is less than the number of moles of reactants.
   C. The phase of the reactants is more ordered than the phase of the product.
   D. The phase of the reactants is more structured than the phase of the product.

18. The heat lost or gained during the breakage and reformation of bonds between atoms in a synthesis reaction is:

   A. Gibbs' free energy.
   B. Helmholtz free energy.
   C. kinetic energy.
   D. heat of reaction.

19. According to Table 2, the formation of CO_2 (g) from elemental carbon and oxygen proceeds spontaneously because:

   A. the reaction produces a net gain in stability.
   B. the reaction produces a net loss in stability.
   C. the reaction produces a net gain in entropy.
   D. the reaction produces a net gain in enthalpy.

20. What is the approximate mass of $FeCl_2$ contained in a 1.0 liter of 0.7 molar solution of $FeCl_2$?

   A. 64 g
   B. 88 g
   C. 130 g
   D. 80 g

21. If a particular synthesis proceeds spontaneously, which of the following should be anticipated?

   A. ΔG is positive; ΔH is negative.
   B. ΔG is positive; ΔH is positive.
   C. ΔG is negative; ΔH is negative.
   D. ΔG is negative; ΔH is positive.

22. When 1 mole of Fe_2O_3 (c) and 1 mole of N_2O_4 (g) are formed from their constituent elements, how much energy is supplied or released to the environment?

   A. 815.0 kJ/mol gained
   B. 815.0 kJ/mol lost
   C. 833.4 kJ/mol gained
   D. 833.4 kJ/mol lost

23. The investigator determined the specific heat of the two compounds, Fe and H_2O. For Fe the value was 0.5 J/g° C, and for H_2O the value was 4.0 J/g° C. If the investigator added 8 g of Fe at 60° C to 99 g of water at 30° C, what would be the temperature of the resulting mixture?

   A. −29.7° C
   B. 0.0° C
   C. 30.3° C
   D. 40.1° C

GO ON TO THE NEXT PAGE

Three common types of radioactive decay are listed below. These processes occur in a fission reactor that uses U-235 as a fuel. Fission of such uranium atoms will occur if they are struck by a high-energy neutron.

Gamma Rays

Gamma rays (γ) are high-energy photons. These particles carry away excess energy when a nuclei moves to a lower energy level. The following reaction is one possible outcome when U-235 is struck by a high-energy neutron.

$$^{235}_{92}U + ^{1}_{0}n \rightarrow ^{92}_{36}Kr + ^{141}_{56}Ba + 2\,^{1}_{0}n + ^{0}_{0}\gamma$$

There are many other massless and chargeless particles that can carry energy away from a nucleus. A neutrino (μ) is such a particle.

Alpha Decay

Some nuclei can spontaneously emit alpha particles ($^{4}_{2}\alpha$). Alpha particles are the nuclei of helium atoms.

A nuclei of U-235 will split when struck by a high-speed neutron. However, this process creates many more high-speed neutrons than it consumes. To keep the reaction from running out of control, most reactors contain control rods made of a material that will absorb the excess neutrons. Boron can be used to absorb high-energy neutrons and instead produce low-energy alpha particles.

$$^{10}_{5}B + ^{1}_{0}n \rightarrow ^{11}_{5}B$$

$$^{11}_{5}B \rightarrow ^{7}_{3}Li + ^{4}_{2}\alpha$$

Beta Decay

A beta particle (β) is an energetic electron. When a nuclei emits a beta particle, it will lose one neutron and gain one proton. Although the probability is very small, U-235 could emit a beta particle and decay to an isotope of neptunium.

$$^{235}_{92}U \rightarrow ^{235}_{93}Np + ^{0}_{-1}\beta$$

(Note: proton mass = 1.0073 amu;
electron rest mass = 9.11×10^{-31} kg;
1 amu = 931 MeV;
1eV = 1.6×10^{-19} J.)

24. Two particles travel through a magnetic field. If the first particle experiences a net force and the second particle is unaffected, which of the following particles are they?

   A. Beta and alpha
   B. Gamma and neutrino
   C. Beta and neutrino
   D. Gamma and alpha

25. Two helium nuclei fuse and release energy in the form of photons. Which of the following describes the main energy transfer that takes place?

   A. Kinetic to kinetic
   B. Electrical to kinetic
   C. Mass to electromagnetic
   D. Kinetic to electrical

26. $^{236}_{90}$Th emits two beta particles and two alpha particles. Which of the following nuclei results?

   A. $^{226}_{87}$Fr

   B. $^{226}_{88}$Ra

   C. $^{228}_{88}$Ra

   D. $^{224}_{86}$Rn

27. Half of a sample of Tl will decay to Pb in 3.1 mins through the emission of beta particles. If an initially pure sample of Tl contains 7 g of lead after 9.3 mins, what was the approximate mass of the original sample?

   A. 7 g
   B. 8 g
   C. 28 g
   D. 32 g

GO ON TO THE NEXT PAGE

28. An element decays to an isotope of itself, releasing alpha and beta particles. The number of alpha particles to beta particles would have to be in the ratio of:

   A. $\dfrac{1}{2}$

   B. 1

   C. 2

   D. 4

29. If 2.8 MeV are needed to produce 1 photon, how many photons can be produced when 1 gram of matter is converted to energy?

   A. 2×10^{26}
   B. 2×10^{32}
   C. 2×10^{35}
   D. 4×10^{35}

Questions 30 through 34 are **NOT** based on a descriptive passage.

30. Light traveling through water in a swimming pool has the following measured values:

   frequency = 5×10^{14} Hz

   phase angle = $\dfrac{\pi}{2}$

   wavelength = 4.5×10^{-7} m

   velocity = 2.25×10^{8} m/s

The wave propagates across the surface of the water into air. If the speed of light in air is 3×10^{8} m/s, what is the frequency of the wave traveling in air?

   A. 2.5×10^{14} Hz
   B. 3.8×10^{14} Hz
   C. 5.0×10^{14} Hz
   D. 6.7×10^{14} Hz

31. A trigonal bipyramid is the characteristic of the orbital geometry of an atom in which hybridization?

   A. sp
   B. sp^2
   C. sp^3
   D. dsp^3

32. Which of the following electronic configurations belongs to a diamagnetic element in its ground state?

   A. $1s^2 2s^1$
   B. $1s^2 2s^2 2p^1$
   C. $1s^2 2s^2 2p^4$
   D. $1s^2 2s^2 2p^6$

33. Three mechanical waves of frequencies 3 Hz, 5 Hz, and 7 Hz are passed through the same medium at equal velocities. The magnitudes of their respective displacement are 1, 2, and 4. What is the smallest possible displacement in the medium that could be caused by the resultant wave?

   A. 0
   B. 1
   C. 7
   D. 8

34. Which of the following is true when comparing Be and Cl?

   A. The electronegativity of Cl is much less than that of Be.
   B. The electron affinity of Cl is much less than that of Be.
   C. The atomic radius of the atom Cl is much larger than that of the atom Be.
   D. Cl is not very reactive, whereas Be, an alkaline Earth metal, is reactive.

GO ON TO THE NEXT PAGE

Passage V (Questions 35–40)

For standard acid-base indicators, the equilibrium reaction is $HIn_A \leftrightarrow H^+ + In_B^-$, where HIn_A is the acid of the indicator with color A, and In_B^- is the conjugate base with color B. Two acid-base indicators are thymol blue (A = red and B = yellow) and bromothymol blue (A = yellow and B = blue).

If an acid is added to an indicator solution, the equilibrium shifts, and color A is produced. Adding a base shifts the equilibrium in the other direction and produces color B.

Acid-base indicators often change color at pH values significantly different from the equivalence points of many titratable acids. Acid-base indicators are most useful for measuring pH changes caused by strong acids such as HCl and H_2SO_4 in aqueous solutions. Near the equivalence point, strong acids exhibit a long, steep rise in their titration curves such that most indicators will change color at some point in this region of the curve. Weaker acids such as acetic acid ($HC_2H_3O_2$) exhibit a much shorter rise. The indicator used with weak acids must change color in a pH range that lies closer to the equivalence point.

A scientist titrated 50 ml of 0.1M HCl with 0.1M NaOH using an unknown acid–base indicator HIn_A. The equivalence point was determined to occur at pH 7.0. A change in color occurred at a pH below the equivalence point.

35. What pH would most likely cause a color change in the unknown indicator?

A. 5
B. 7
C. 9
D. 14

36. Which of the following colors would result from the formation of the conjugate base of bromothymol blue?

A. Spectral red
B. Blue
C. Yellow
D. Green

37. At pH 7.0, the solution's color most probably indicates the presence of:

A. HIn_A
B. In_A^-
C. In_B^-
D. HIn_B^-

38. Two additional indicators were used. For HCl, phenolphthalein changed color above the equivalence point, and methyl red changed color below the equivalence point. At the equivalence point, which forms of the indicators produce color?

A. The base of phenolphthalein and the acid of methyl red
B. The base of methyl red and the acid of phenolphthalein
C. The acids of both indicators
D. The bases of both indicators

39. The color change of the unknown indicator represented a shift of the equilibrium reaction $HIn_A \leftrightarrow H^+ + In_B^-$:

A. to the ground state configuration.
B. to formation of the conjugate acid.
C. to the left.
D. to the right.

40. According to the information presented below, which of the following indicators will be present in the acid form in an aqueous titration solution that reached pH 5.0?

Indicator	Acid	Base Color	$K_{ind,}$ Color	pH Range
Thymol blue	Red	Yellow	2×10^{-2}	1.2 – 2.8
Methyl orange	Red	Orange	3.5×10^{-4}	3.1 – 4.4
Bromothymol blue	Yellow	Blue	8×10^{-8}	6.0 – 7.6

A. Thymol blue, because the conjugate acid remains protonated at the pH value of the solution
B. Thymol blue, because the conjugate base is deprotonated at the pH value of the solution
C. Bromothymol blue, because the conjugate acid remains protonated at the pH value of the solution
D. Bromothymol blue, because the conjugate base is deprotonated at the pH value of the solution

GO ON TO THE NEXT PAGE

60 CRACKING THE MCAT

A U-shaped glass tube has a diameter of 0.1 m and is filled with a liquid of density 5.0×10^3 kg/m^3. The liquid settles to a height of h_0 in both stems A and B. A piston of negligible mass is then fitted into stem A of the tube, forming a perfect seal. By moving the piston up or down, work is done by or on the fluid according to the following equation:

$$W = (P_i - P_f) \; \triangle V$$

where P_i and P_f are the initial and final pressures on the fluid, and V is the displaced volume of fluid in stem A.
(Note: Assume that the density of the fluid remains constant.)

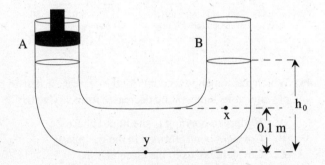

41. The piston is pulled upward so that the new fluid heights in stems A and B are h_1 and h_2 respectively. Which of the following relate h_0, h_1, and h_2?

   A. $h_0 < h_1 < h_2$
   B. $h_1 < h_0 < h_2$
   C. $h_2 < h_0 < h_1$
   D. $h_0 = h_2 < h_1$

42. If both stems A and B have fluid at height h_0, what is the difference in pressure between points x and y? (Assume atmospheric pressure is 1.013×10^5 Pa.)

   A. 5.0×10^3 Pa
   B. 1.0×10^5 Pa
   C. 1.5×10^5 Pa
   D. 2.5×10^5 Pa

43. If the piston is moved such that the height of the fluid in stem A is lowered by 20% of its initial height, h_0, what is the work done on the fluid in terms of h_0 and π? (Use 10 m/s^2 for the value of gravitational acceleration.)

   A. $\dfrac{\pi(h_0)}{10}$ J

   B. $5\pi (h_0)^2$ J

   C. $2\pi \times 10^7 \, h_0$ J

   D. $\dfrac{25\pi \times 10^5}{h_0}$ J

44. The piston is removed and the liquid reaches a height of 20 m in each stem. A small hole appears at point y, and a steady flow of fluid escapes. Ignoring friction, what is the velocity at which fluid leaves the U-tube? (Use 10 m/s^2 for the value of gravitational acceleration.)

   A. 10 m/s
   B. 12 m/s
   C. 17 m/s
   D. 20 m/s

GO ON TO THE NEXT PAGE

The phase-related properties of water have been subjected to considerable scientific scrutiny. The table below lists several of these properties.

Property	Properties of Water
Density	0.99707 g/cm³ at 25° C * 1.00000 g/cm³ at 4° C 0.99987 g/cm³ at 0° C
Heat of Fusion	6.008 kJ/mol at 0° C
Heat of Vaporization	44.02 kJ/mol at 25° C 44.94 kJ/mol at 0° C
Vapor Pressure	23.76 mm Hg at 25° C ** 6.54 mm Hg at 5° C 4.58 mm Hg at 0° C

* Density decreases as temperature rises above 25° C.
** Vapor pressure increases as temperature rises above 25° C.

Water in the solid phase has an open lattice structure which is facilitated by the extensive amount of hydrogen bonding within the lattice.

In the liquid phase, water demonstrates decreasing cohesive forces upon heating. For example, when water is heated from 20° C to 60° C, the viscosity of water decreases more than 50 percent while the surface tension decreases approximately 5 percent. This trend continues at higher temperatures.

Water vapor pressure contributes to the total pressure of a gaseous mixture collected over water. At 0° C, water vapor contributes 4.58 mm Hg to the total pressure of the mixture. Near 100° C, the water vapor contribution to total gas pressure approaches 760 mm Hg.

45. The dependence of the viscosity and surface tension of water on temperature is best illustrated by which of the following figures?

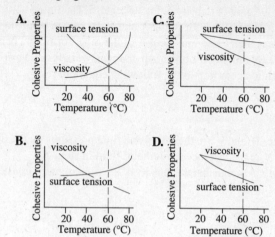

46. Which phenomenon accounts for the decrease in density of water as its temperature decreases from 4 °C to 0 °C?

A. Hydrogen bonding in the liquid phase
B. Covalent bonds formed in the gas phase
C. Covalent bonds in the closed lattice
D. Hydrogen bonding in the open lattice

47. When ice melts at 0° C, what enthalpy change occurs during the formation of the liquid phase under standard equilibrium conditions?

A. The reaction releases 6.008 kJ/mol.
B. The reaction consumes 6.008 kJ/mol.
C. The reaction releases 44.02 kJ/mol.
D. The reaction equilibrium results in 44.94 kJ/mol energy release.

GO ON TO THE NEXT PAGE

48. A water molecule is able to form hydrogen bonds because of its:

   A. ability to form a crystalline lattice at vaporization.
   B. ability to form ionic bonds, as measured by ionization energy.
   C. ability to form covalent bonds, as measured by its electron affinity.
   D. degree of polarity, as measured by the dipole moment.

49. The volume of 1.00 g of water at 4° C under standard pressures is less than the volume of 1.00 g of water at 25° C.

   These results confirm that water at 25° C:

   A. has a lower density.
   B. has a higher vapor pressure.
   C. has a greater molecular weight.
   D. undergoes ionization.

50. The hybrid orbitals in a water molecule are correctly identified by which of the following?

   A. 4 sp^3 orbitals in a trigonal array with two nonbonding pairs of electrons
   B. 4 sp^3 orbitals in a tetrahedral array with two nonbonding pairs of electrons
   C. 4 sp^2 orbitals in a trigonal array with two nonbonding pairs of electrons
   D. 3 sp^2 orbitals in a tetrahedral array with three nonbonding pairs of electrons

Questions 51 through 55 are **NOT** based on a descriptive passage.

51. Within the orbital structure of an atom, as the second quantum number (l) increases, the number of orbitals:

   A. increases according to $2l$.
   B. increases according to $2l + 1$.
   C. increases according to l.
   D. remains the same.

52. A car of mass m is rolling down a ramp that is elevated at an angle of 60°. What is the magnitude of the car's acceleration parallel to the ramp?

   A. $\dfrac{mg\sqrt{3}}{3}$

   B. $\dfrac{\sqrt{3}g}{2}$

   C. $\dfrac{g}{2}$

   D. $\dfrac{2g}{3}$

53. When an electron is added to a neutral atom to form its anion, the atomic radius:

   A. decreases, because the added electron makes the orbital more complete.
   B. increases, because the effective nuclear charge decreases.
   C. increases, because the electronegativity of the atom decreases.
   D. stays the same, because the added electron contributes negligible mass to the atom.

GO ON TO THE NEXT PAGE

54. Two sinusoidal waves, one with a frequency of 14 cycles per minute, the other with a frequency of 12 cycles per minute, are sent down a rope. The frequency of the combined wave is:

    A. 14 cycles/min.
    B. 26 cycles/min.
    C. 84 cycles/min.
    D. 168 cycles/min.

55. The atomic radius of $_{11}^{22}\text{Na}$ is approximately twice that of $_{18}^{40}\text{Ar}$, mainly because:

    A. the ionization energy of Ar is greater than that of Na.
    B. Ar is inert, whereas Na easily forms an ion.
    C. the valence electrons of Na are more effectively shielded from the nucleus than the valence electrons of Ar.
    D. Ar has 18 protons attracting its electrons, whereas Na has only 11 protons.

Passage VIII (Questions 56–61)

A hollow tube with one closed end can be used to set up a standing sound wave. A standing wave will form if the length of the tube is an odd-integer multiple of one-quarter the wavelength of the sound entering the tube. When a standing wave forms, the column of air inside the tube is said to resonate. Almost all musical instruments work on this principle. For example, a guitar player produces different notes by changing the frequencies at which the strings on his instrument resonate.

The apparatus depicted in the figure below exploits the phenomenon of resonance to calculate the speed of sound. The water level in the tube can be lowered by releasing water through the valve located near the bottom. Lowering the water level effectively lengthens the tube. The tuning fork is struck and held near the open end of the tube. The tuning fork emits sound waves at 440 Hz. As the water level is lowered, it is observed that the air in the tube resonates at multiples of a fixed length.

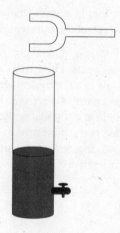

56. Approximately what is the period of the wave produced by the tuning fork?

    A. .0007 s
    B. .0023 s
    C. .0071 s
    D. .0440 s

GO ON TO THE NEXT PAGE

57. Which of the following figures best represents a standing sound wave inside the tube?

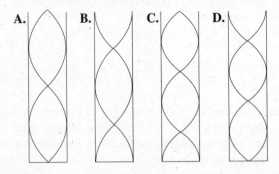

A.   B.   C.   D.

58. If the tube's diameter were increased, which of the following would be true regarding the period and/or frequency of the standing wave inside it?

A. Its wavelength would increase.
B. Its wavelength would decrease.
C. Its period would increase.
D. Its wavelength and period would remain unchanged.

59. As the water level in the tube is lowered, resonance occurs at intervals of .37 m. This implies that the speed of sound in air is:

A. 163 m/s.
B. 326 m/s.
C. 330 m/s.
D. 370 m/s.

60. The room in which the experiment takes place is filled with helium. The density of helium gas is much less than that of air. What changes will occur to the standing wave?

A. The distance between antinodes will increase.
B. The distance between antinodes will decrease.
C. The distance between antinodes will remain the same.
D. No standing wave will form.

61. Which of the following would indicate that the tuning fork was rapidly moving away from the end of the tube?

A. The amplitude of the sound waves reaching the tube is greater than expected.
B. The amplitude of the sound waves reaching the tube is less than expected.
C. The frequency of the sound waves reaching the tube is greater than expected.
D. The frequency of the sound waves reaching the tube is less than expected.

GO ON TO THE NEXT PAGE

Passage IX (Questions 62–67)

In studying the properties of gases, scientists often employ the ideal gas equation, $PV = nRT$. In this equation, n represents the number of moles of the gas present.

If n increases while T is held constant, the quantity PV will increase. If pressure and temperature are held constant, volume must increase to satisfy the ideal gas equation. Similarly, if temperature and volume are held constant if n increases, pressure must also increase. Figure 1 represents the relationship between n and PV while temperature is held constant.

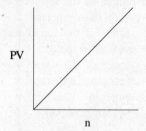

Figure 1

Scientists and engineers often work with gases at high pressures. Gases under these conditions show large departures from the ideal gas equation. The equation could better model gases at high pressures if P is substituted with $P + (an^2/V^2)$, and V is substituted with $V-nb$. The constants a and b are van der Waals constants. The values of PV/RT in terms of pressure for nitrogen and hydrogen gases at 300 K are shown in Figure 2. The dotted line plots values predicted by the ideal gas law.

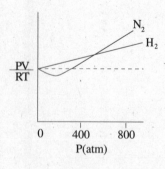

Figure 2

In reality, the value used for V should be the volume of the container less the total space occupied by the molecules. Under normal circumstances, the space taken up by the molecules is insignificant. However, under high–pressure situations, the volume correction must be taken into account. This fact is the primary cause for the deviation between the predicted and observed results in Figure 2.

Substance	Constant a	Constant b
Helium	0.0341	0.02370
Neon	0.211	0.0171
H_2	0.244	0.0266
N_2	1.39	0.0391
Cl_2	6.49	0.0562

62. If the number of moles of a gas in a 1 liter container is decreased at 300 K, which of the following figures best represents the relationship between the number of moles and pressure?

A.

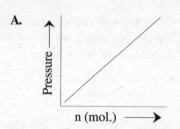

B.

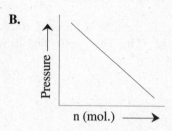

C.

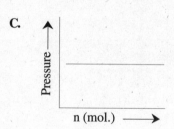

D.

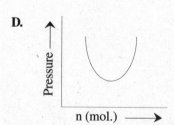

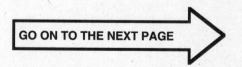

GO ON TO THE NEXT PAGE

63. A researcher wishes to compare real gas behavior to gas behavior predicted by the ideal gas law. The researcher subjects a gas sample to relatively high pressure and then compares the pressure actually measured to that which would be predicted according to the ideal gas law. The pressure *actually measured* is probably:

  A. greater than that predicted by the ideal gas law because of repulsive forces among gas particles.
  B. greater than that predicted by the ideal gas law because of attractive forces among gas particles.
  C. less than that predicted by the ideal gas law because of repulsive forces among gas particles.
  D. less than that predicted by the ideal gas law because of attractive forces among gas particles.

64. A decrease in the number of moles of a gas at constant temperature and volume will decrease which of the following unit measures?

  A. Cubic centimeters
  B. Number of atoms per cm^3
  C. Joules per mole of gas
  D. Cubic centimeters occupied by the gas

65. Which of the following will demonstrate a greater departure from the behavior of an ideal gas: hydrogen gas or helium gas?

  A. Helium gas, because the van der Waals corrections are lower than for hydrogen.
  B. Helium gas, because it is an inert gas.
  C. Hydrogen gas, because the van der Waals corrections are greater than for helium.
  D. Hydrogen gas, because hydrogen shows decreased intermolecular forces at higher pressures.

66. Which of the following best illustrates the values of PV/RT in terms of pressure for hydrogen gas and a second gas, A_2, that shows greater compression at high pressures? (Note: The dotted line represents the values of PV/RT for an ideal gas under high pressures.)

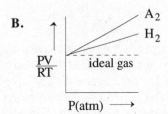

B.

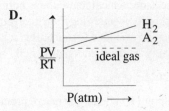

67. From the passage above, what would be the van der Waals correction for the volume (cm^3) for 2 moles of neon gas at pressures over 400 atm?

  A. $V - 0.02370$
  B. $V - 0.0391$
  C. $V - 2 \times 0.02370$
  D. $V - 2 \times 0.0171$

GO ON TO THE NEXT PAGE

Passage X (Questions 68–73)

The prototypical astronomical telescope is designed as shown in Figure 1 below.

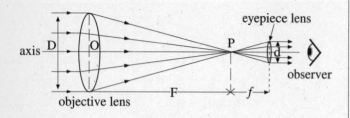

Figure 1

The objective lens, O, has a long positive focal length. The incident parallel rays emanating from the object to be visualized enter from the left and traverse the objective lens which has diameter D. The eyepiece is located nearer the observer. It has a short positive focal length and acts as a magnifying glass.

The focal lengths F and f of the objective lens and eyepiece respectively coincide at point P, the site of an image that is real and inverted. The image at point P directs light rays to the eyepiece which transforms it into an enlarged virtual image that remains inverted. The inversion is of little practical consequence because the astronomical telescope is normally used to study distant objects. Rays emerging from the eyepiece embody all of the information available for the observer's eye and are known collectively as the "emergent pencil," with diameter d.

68. For an observer at point P viewing the image produced by the objective lens, the observer would see an image at:

A. $\frac{F}{4}$.

B. $\frac{F}{2}$.

C. the surface of the objective lens.

D. negative infinity.

69. Assuming that the incident parallel rays enter the objective lens at a small angle θ to the axis of the telescope, which of the following figures shows a possible path for the light rays? (Some dimensions have been distorted for clarity.)

A.

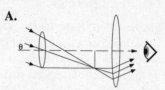

B.

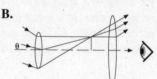

C.

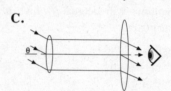

D.

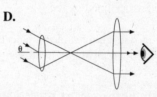

70. With reference to the observer depicted in Figure 1, which of the following statements applies to the image at point P?

A. It serves as an object for the eyepiece.
B. It serves as an object for the objective lens.
C. It is real and upright.
D. It is virtual and inverted.

GO ON TO THE NEXT PAGE

71. The two lenses in Figure 1 act together as a single equivalent lens with a focal length of:

- **A.** $F + f$.
- **B.** $F \times f$.
- **C.** $\dfrac{Ff}{F + f}$.
- **D.** $\dfrac{F + f}{Ff}$.

72. If the observer is viewing a comet that is moving toward the telescope, how will the image seen by the observer differ from one of a stationary body?

- **A.** The color of the image corresponds to that of a lower frequency.
- **B.** The color of the image corresponds to that of a higher frequency.
- **C.** The image will be brighter.
- **D.** The image will be more blurred.

73. Referring to the light rays drawn in Figure 1, which of the following is true?

- **A.** The objective lens is a diverging lens.
- **B.** The eyepiece lens is a diverging lens.
- **C.** Both lenses are converging lenses.
- **D.** Both lenses are diverging lenses.

74. Based on the table below, which of the following species is the weakest oxidizing agent?

Half-Reaction	Standard Potential
$Br_2(l) + 2e^- \rightarrow 2Br^-(aq)$	1.08
$Ag_2O(s) + H_2O + 2e \rightarrow 2Ag(s) + 2OH^-(aq)$	0.34
$Cu^{2+}(aq) + e^- \rightarrow Cu^+(aq)$	0.15
$H_2(g) + 2e^- \rightarrow 2H^-(aq)$	0.00

   A. H_2
   B. Cu^{2+}
   C. Br_2
   D. Ag_2O

75. An atom is in its ground state with all the orbitals filled through n = 2 main energy level. How many electrons are contained in this atom?

   A. 8
   B. 10
   C. 12
   D. 14

76. A uranium-238 nucleus emits an alpha particle (helium nucleus) and decays to thorium-234. The alpha particle leaves the nucleus traveling 4.68×10^5 m/s. At what speed would the thorium nucleus recoil? (Note: Assume the masses of a proton and a neutron are equal.)

   A. 1.5×10^3 m/s
   B. 4.0×10^3 m/s
   C. 8.0×10^3 m/s
   D. 2.5×10^4 m/s

77. The half-life of material X is 1 min. The half-life of material Y is three times greater than that of material X. Starting with 1 g samples of X and Y, how much more of material X would have decayed after 6 min?

   A. $\dfrac{7}{32}$ g

   B. $\dfrac{15}{64}$ g

   C. $\dfrac{3}{8}$ g

   D. 2 g

STOP
IF YOU FINISH BEFORE TIME IS CALLED, YOU MAY CHECK YOUR WORK ON THIS TEST ONLY.
DO NOT TURN TO ANY OTHER TEST IN THIS BOOK.

Writing Sample

Time: 60 Minutes
2 Prompts, Separately Timed:
30 Minutes Each

WRITING SAMPLE: EXPLANATIONS

The following essays were written according to The Princeton Review's MCAT Essay Formula. As described in Part I, they are designed to make a "good impression" on a reader who will spend approximately *ninety seconds* evaluating them. Notice that each essay:

1. performs, in appropriate order, all three "tasks" described in the MCAT instructions,

2. provides frequent paragraphing,

3. uses formal language, and—

4. cites a quotation from some famed authority.

WRITING SAMPLE

DIRECTIONS: This is a test of your writing skills. The test consists of two parts. You will have 30 minutes to complete each part.

Your responses to the Writing Sample prompts will be written in ANSWER DOCUMENT 2. Your response to Part 1 must be written only on the answer sheets marked "1," and your response to Part 2 must be written only on the answer sheets marked "2." You may work only on Part 1 during the first 30 minutes of the test and only on Part 2 during the second 30 minutes. If you finish writing on Part 1 before time is up, you may review your work on that part, but do not begin work on Part 2. If you finish writing on Part 2 before time is up, you may review your work only on that part of the test.

Use your time efficiently. Before you begin writing each of your responses, read the assignment carefully to understand exactly what you are being asked to do. You may use the space beneath each writing assignment to make notes in planning each response.

Because this is a test of your writing skills, your response to each part should be an essay of complete sentences and paragraphs, as well organized and clearly written as you can make it in the allotted time. *You may make corrections or additions neatly between the lines of your responses, but do not write in the margins of the answer booklet.*

There are six pages in your answer booklet to write your responses, three pages for each part of the test. You are not expected to use all of the pages, but to ensure that you have enough room for each essay, do not skip lines.

Essays that are illegible cannot be scored.

Part 1

Consider this statement:

People get the government they deserve.

Write a unified essay in which you perform the following tasks: Explain what you think the above statement means. Describe a specific situation in which people do not get the government they deserve. Discuss what you think determines whether or not people get the government they deserve.

Part 2

Consider this statement:

Honesty is essential to friendship.

Write a unified essay in which you perform the following tasks: Explain what you think the above statement means. Describe a specific situation in which honesty is not essential to friendship. Discuss what you think determines whether or not honesty is essential to friendship.

STOP
THIS IS THE END OF SECTION 3. DO NOT RETURN TO PART 1.

Biological Sciences

Time: 100 Minutes

Questions 1–77

DIRECTIONS: Most questions in the Biological Sciences test are organized into groups, each preceded by a descriptive passage. After studying the passage, select the one best answer to each question in the group. Some questions are not based on a descriptive passage and are also independent of each other. You must also select the one best answer to these questions. If you are not certain of an answer, eliminate the alternatives that you know to be incorrect and then select an answer from the remaining alternatives. Indicate your selection by blackening the corresponding circle on your answer sheet (DIAGNOSTIC TEST FORM). A periodic table is provided for your use. You may consult it whenever you wish.

PERIODIC TABLE OF THE ELEMENTS

1 H 1.0																	2 He 4.0
3 Li 6.9	4 Be 9.0											5 B 10.8	6 C 12	2 N 14.0	8 O 16	9 F 19.0	10 Ne 20.0
11 Na 22.0	12 Mg 24.3											13 Al 27.0	14 Si 28.1	15 P 31.0	16 S 32.1	17 Cl 35.5	18 Ar 39.0
19 K 39.1	20 Ca 40.1	21 Sc 45.0	22 Ti 47.9	23 V 50.9	24 Cr 52.0	25 Mn 54.9	26 Fe 55.8	27 Co 58.9	28 Ni 58.7	29 Cu 63.5	30 Zn 65.4	31 Ga 69.7	32 Ge 72.6	33 As 74.9	34 Se 79.0	35 Br 79.9	36 Kr 83.8
37 Rb 85.5	38 Sr 87.6	39 Y 88.9	40 Zr 91.2	41 Nb 92.9	42 Mo 95.9	43 Tc 97.0	44 Ru 101.0	45 Rh 102.9	46 Pd 106.4	47 Ag 107.9	48 Cd 112.4	49 In 114.8	50 Sn 118.7	51 Sb 121.8	52 Te 127.6	53 I 126.9	54 Xe 131.3
55 Cs 132.9	56 Ba 137.3	57 La 138.9	72 Hf 178.5	73 Ta 180.9	74 W 183.9	75 Re 186.2	76 Os 190.2	77 Ir 192.2	78 Pt 195.1	79 Au 197.0	80 Hg 200.6	81 Tl 204.4	82 Pb 207.2	83 Bi 209.0	84 Po 209.0	85 At 210.0	86 Rn 222.0
87 Fr 223.0	88 Ra 226.0	89 Ac 227.0															

58 Ce 140.1	59 Pr 140.9	60 Nd 144.2	61 Pm 145.0	62 Sm 150.4	63 Eu 152.0	64 Gd 157.3	65 Tb 158.9	66 Dy 162.5	67 Ho 164.9	68 Er 167.3	69 Tm 168.9	70 Yb 173.0	71 Lu 175.0
90 Th 232.0	91 Pa 231.0	92 U 238.0	93 Np 237.0	94 Pu 244.0	95 Am 243.0	96 Cm 247.0	97 Bk 247.0	98 Cf 251.0	99 Es 254.0	100 Fm 253.0	101 Md 256.0	102 No 253.0	103 Lr 257.0

Passage I (Questions 1–6)

Within animals that have closed circulatory systems, the space that lies both outside the cells of the body and outside the circulatory system is called the interstitial compartment. This compartment normally has fluid in it. The precise volume of this fluid represents a balance between two factors.

The first of these factors is the *fluid pressure* within the blood vessels, which tends to force fluid out of the vessels and into the interstitial space. The second factor is the *colloid pressure,* which is created by the higher levels of protein in the blood as compared with the interstitial space. Blood vessels have higher protein levels than the interstitial compartment because the vessels are not normally permeable to protein. The difference in protein levels creates a gradient that tends to draw fluid into the vessels from the interstitial space.

The role of colloid pressure in determining interstitial fluid volume has been studied through a technique in which (1) the circulatory system of an animal cadaver is opened at the arterial end and at the venous end, and (2) fluid is pumped in through the arterial opening and through the vasculature, and then drained out at the venous opening.

Experiment 1

The circulatory systems of three 60 kg animal cadavers were infused with fluids having different protein concentrations, according to the technique described above. Cadaver A received fluid with the lowest protein concentration, and Cadaver C received fluid with the highest concentration. At ten-minute intervals, the cadavers were weighed to determine how much interstitial fluid had been drawn into the circulatory system and drained through the venous opening. The infused fluid was also weighed.

The results are tabulated in Table 1.

Infusion Time	Body Weight		
	Cadaver A	Cadaver B	Cadaver C
10 min.	60 kg	60 kg	60 kg
20 min.	53 kg	47 kg	36 kg
30 min.	44 kg	32 kg	28 kg
40 min.	31 kg	23 kg	27 kg
50 min.	24 kg	23 kg	27 kg
60 min.	24 kg	23 kg	27 kg
70 min.	24 kg	23 kg	27 kg

Table 1

Experiment 2

The circulatory system of one 75 kg cadaver—Cadaver D—was infused with fluid lacking any protein, according to the same technique described above. The cadaver was weighed at ten-minute intervals. The results are tabulated in Table 2.

Infusion Time	Body Weight
	Cadaver D
10 min.	75 kg
20 min.	75 kg
30 min.	75 kg
40 min.	75 kg
50 min.	75 kg
60 min.	75 kg
70 min.	75 kg

Table 2

1. In humans, the peptide bonds of ingested proteins are first cleaved in the stomach by which of the following enzymes?

   A. Lactase
   B. Pepsin
   C. Amylase
   D. Lipase

2. Colloid pressure tends to draw fluid into the blood vessels by:

   A. passive diffusion along a concentration gradient.
   B. passive diffusion along an electrical gradient.
   C. facilitated transport along an electrochemical gradient.
   D. active diffusion, mediated by an ATP-dependent pump.

GO ON TO THE NEXT PAGE

3. A professor theorized that if a patient's capillaries became suddenly permeable to protein, the patient would manifest edema. Is this a plausible hypothesis?

A. No, fluid will move across a membrane only in response to an ion gradient.

B. No, protein permeability would have no effect on hydrostatic pressure within the blood vessel.

C. Yes, protein would fuel the active transport of fluid into the interstitial space.

D. Yes, colloid pressure would decrease, and fluid would leak into the interstitial space.

4. The blood proteins that produce colloid pressure are synthesized by a sequential mechanism that involves the direct activity of:

A. cellular proteases.

B. smooth endoplasmic reticulum.

C. messenger RNA.

D. cytochromes.

5. Given the results of Experiments 1 and 2, a researcher would be most justified in concluding that:

A. Cadaver D had a higher protein concentration in its interstitial fluid than did Cadavers A, B, or C.

B. Cadaver A contained more interstitial fluid than did Cadaver B, which contained more interstitial fluid than did Cadaver C.

C. Cadavers A, B, and C were composed of at least 50 percent interstitial fluid by weight.

D. Cadaver C was composed of approximately 80 percent interstitial fluid by weight.

6. If, in a normal patient, proteins were suddenly infused into the interstitial space, which of the following physiological compensations could prevent the resulting edema?

A. Reduction of hydrostatic pressure within the blood vessels

B. Passive diffusion of proteins from the blood vessels to the interstitial space

C. Facilitated diffusion of protein from the blood vessels to the interstitial space

D. Increase in protein synthesis by the red blood cells

Passage II (Questions 7–13)

Metabolism is the process that organisms utilize to derive free energy from the oxidation of fuel molecules. In eukaryotic cells, metabolism includes the process of oxidative phosphorylation. This process occurs on the mitochondrial respiratory chain and forms ATP by transferring electrons from NADH and $FADH_2$ to oxygen. The mitochondrial respiratory chain, with inhibitors, is illustrated in Figure 1.

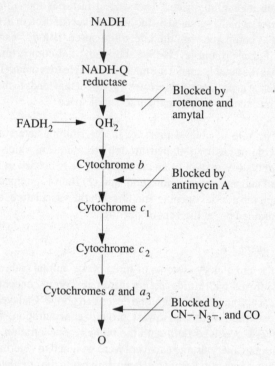

Figure 1

To elucidate the site inhibited by Antimycin A, an antibiotic, researchers carried out the following protocols:

• Mitochondrial extracts with normal respiratory chains were exposed to Antimycin A in the presence of NADH and $FADH_2$.

• Oxygen consumption before and after antibiotic administration was measured, and mitochondrial cytochrome structure was analyzed by X-ray crystallography.

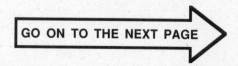

It was found that the inhibited structure was cytochrome b, which possesses the heme-containing center pictured in Figure 2.

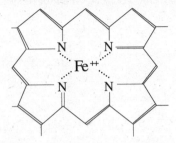

Figure 2

There was a significant drop in oxygen consumption upon administration of Antimycin A.

7. When concluding that the drop in oxygen consumption is due only to inhibition of cytochrome b, the researchers most probably assumed that Antimycin A:

    A. increases levels of CO_2.
    B. decreases levels of oxygen in the atmosphere.
    C. attacks only the respiratory chain.
    D. attacks other oxidative mitochondrial enzymes.

8. Which of the following phosphorous-containing compounds can circumvent the effects of rotenone, as seen in Figure 1?

    A. $FADH_2$ circumvents the effects of rotenone.
    B. Both NADH and ADP circumvent the inhibition.
    C. Both NADH and ADP circumvent the inhibition; $FADH_2$ also circumvents the effects of rotenone, but it does not contain phosphorous.
    D. $FADH_2$, NADH, and ADP circumvent the inhibition of NADH dehydrogenase by rotenone.

9. Aerobic organisms generate the greatest number of ATPs when monosaccharide oxidation produces:

    A. reduced levels of anti-oxidants.
    B. reduced forms of NAD^+ and FAD.
    C. oxidized forms of ATP and GTP.
    D. oxidized forms of NADH and $FADH_2$.

10. A substance that inhibits NADH-Q reductase will have little effect if the cell is adequately supplied with which phosphorous-containing compound?

    A. $FADH_2$
    B. NADPH
    C. ADP
    D. NADH

11. The presence of fully functioning respiratory chains in the mitochondrial extracts was vital to the success of the experiment. If cytochrome c_1 had been missing, the researcher most likely would have found that:

    A. extra cytochrome c_1 had accumulated.
    B. NADH and $FADH_2$ could not enter the system.
    C. Antimycin A had increased oxygen consumption.
    D. Antimycin A had had no effect.

12. To further characterize cytochrome b, the researchers reacted its sulfur-containing amino acids with performic acid and then broke apart the polypeptide into individual amino acid residues. The most likely means of performing this latter task is to:

    A. reduce cysteine residues.
    B. decarboxylate acidic residues.
    C. oxidize amide linkages.
    D. hydrolyze amide linkages.

13. The heme portions of cytochrome molecules are able to transfer electrons among themselves because of:

    A. thioether linkages.
    B. pi-electron delocalization.
    C. enol-intermediate racemization.
    D. shortened bond length.

GO ON TO THE NEXT PAGE

Passage III (Questions 14–18)

A milk inspector was sent by the state Food and Drug Administration to a dairy plant to randomly sample containers of both raw and pasteurized milk to certify that milk production was being conducted under sanitary conditions. Milk contamination may be the result of several types of bacterial growth. The first organism to flourish in milk is usually *Streptococcuslactis,* which ferments the sugar lactose to lactic acid. The chemical environment produced by fermentation is conducive to the growth of the nonsporeforming, gram-positive organism *Lactobacillus,* which then predominates. Facultative anaerobic, sporeforming bacteria such as *Streptococcus faecalis* may also be present. Fresh milk that contains emulsified fat droplets tends to be anaerobic and has a pH of about 7. Pasteurization is the most common procedure that kills nonsporeforming pathogenic bacteria. The FDA's laboratory conducted the examination according to the procedure below:

1. Take 10 samples of raw and pasteurized milk.
2. Shake each sample vigorously to obtain a homogeneous sample of milk.
3. Using a pipette, transfer 10 mls of each sample of milk to 20 sterilized test tubes.
4. Heat the tubes and hold at 50° C for 15 minutes in a water bath and then add sufficient melted vaspar to form a 1/2-inch layer on the milk in each tube.
5. Incubate all tubes at 37° C for at least 3 days.
6. Make thin smears and stain with methylene blue and gram stain.

14. Which of the following best describes the appearance of *Lactobacillus* when stained and then viewed with a light microscope?

   A. Spherical
   B. S-shaped
   C. Rodlike
   D. Asymmetrical

15. The proliferation of *Lactobacillus* in milk samples indicates:

   A. high lactose concentration.
   B. a drop in the pH.
   C. predominance of sporeforming bacteria.
   D. the absence of *Streptococcus faecalis.*

16. If one of the raw milk samples were heated to 100°C for 30 minutes, the graph of sporeforming and nonsporeforming bacteria would be which of the following?

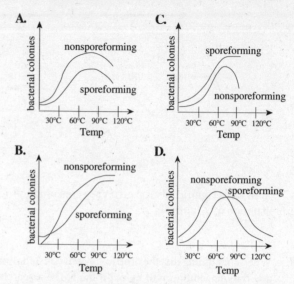

17. The gram-staining procedure used in the laboratory enables the inspector to:

   A. identify bacterial species present in the incubate.
   B. distinguish between aerobic and anaerobic organisms.
   C. differentiate pathogenic from nonpathogenic colonies.
   D. distinguish between bacterial and viral organisms.

18. Which of the following environmental factors will affect the growth of *S. faecalis*?

   I. Nutritional content of the milk
   II. The process of pasteurization
   III. Ambient oxygen concentration

   A. I only
   B. I and II
   C. I and III
   D. I, II, and III

GO ON TO THE NEXT PAGE

19. The *eclipsed* conformation of *n*-butane is illustrated below, in the figure on the left. Which of the circled positions in the figure on the right corresponds to the terminal methyl group in the *anti* conformation?

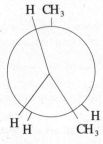 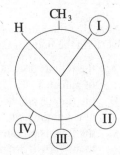

A. I
B. II
C. III
D. IV

20. All of the following structures secrete enzymes that serve digestive functions EXCEPT:

A. pancreas.
B. stomach.
C. thymus.
D. mouth.

21. Alkyl halides are more reactive than their corresponding alkanes because the halides more readily participate in:

A. pyrolysis.
B. combustion reactions.
C. hydrophobic bonding.
D. nucleophilic substitution.

22. When lettuce is placed in deionized water it remains crisp because:

A. the cells lose H_2O.
B. the cells swell with H_2O.
C. the stomates close in response to excess water.
D. the chloroplasts generate greater levels of ATP.

23. Among the following, which statements can be said to apply to the hypothetical molecule depicted schematically below?

I. It rotates the plane of polarized light to the left
II. It exhibits chirality
III. It is optically active

A. I only
B. I and II only
C. I and III only
D. II and III only

24. Which statement below most accurately describes the characteristic features of striated muscle cells?

A. Striated muscle cells are stimulated by the autonomic nervous system and contain few mitochondria.
B. Striated muscle cells are mononucleate and arranged in syncytial bundles.
C. Striated muscle cells have alternating A-bands and I-bands arranged in a transverse pattern.
D. Striated muscle cells are similar to smooth muscle cells except they lack internal stores of calcium.

GO ON TO THE NEXT PAGE

Passage IV (Questions 25–29)

Invasive candidiasis is a disease in humans that is caused by several members of the fungal Candida species, including *Candida albicans* and *Candida tropicalis*. Candida are easily detected in tissue samples because of their sturdy cell walls, which contain polysaccharides and ergosterol.

In pathological circumstances, Candida are found both in the unicellular yeast form and the multicellular, nonbranching pseudohyphal form. In the yeast form, Candida divide by asexual budding, which involves replication of DNA by mitosis without the formation of germ cells. The pseudohyphal form grows in nonbranching strands and reproduces mostly by asexual budding. However, the pseudohypha can also form fruiting bodies that produce gametes (spores). These spores are haploid and can fuse to form a diploid zygote. Both the yeast and pseudohyphal forms of Candida can invade many different organ systems via the bloodstream.

All of the following drugs have been used in the treatment of Candidal infections. These drugs either attack the fungal cell wall or interfere with replication or transcription.

1. Amphotericin B binds to ergosterol in the outer membrane and increases fungal cell wall permeability and damage.

2. Ketoconazole is a compound that interferes with ergosterol synthesis, and thus also increases cell wall permeability.

3. 5-Fluorocytosine (5-FC) is a synthetic pyrimidine that interferes with the synthesis of RNA in fungal cells.

5-FC is deaminated by fungal cells to yield 5-fluorouracil (5-FU). An intermediate product of 5-FU binds to the enzyme thymidylate synthetase, blocking its ability to catalyze the formation of thymidine. The structure of 5-FC is shown below.

25. Which of the following treatments would NOT be an effective means of treating Candidal infections?

A. Administration of a drug that attacks the outer cell wall of the fungus
B. Administration of a drug that interferes with fungal replication and transcription
C. Exposure to the infective form of the fungus itself
D. Exposure to oral fungistatic drugs

26. Attacking the gamete-producing stage of Candida does NOT rid the body of Candidal infection because:

A. the fungus does not reproduce by the formation of gametes.
B. the fungus can be killed only by using drugs that also kill the host.
C. the fungus produces gametes that are insensitive to all known drugs.
D. the fungus is most often in a form that reproduces asexually.

27. 5-FC attacks the Candida fungus by decreasing:

A. the need for formation of gametes.
B. the availability of DNA and RNA precursors.
C. the availability of necessary amino acids.
D. the availability of 5-FU.

28. After absorption of 5-FC, which next step must occur for 5-FC to terminate DNA synthesis?

A. One pyrimidine is substituted for another pyrimidine.
B. A purine must be converted into a pyrimidine.
C. Uracil must be converted into thymidine.
D. Thymidylate synthetase must be phosphorylated to be inactivated.

GO ON TO THE NEXT PAGE

29. When undergoing reproduction, the predominant form of Candida in the human body according to the passage maintains:

A. the same number of chromosomes per nucleus, while randomly dividing the genome between two daughter cells.

B. the same number of chromosomes per nucleus, without randomly dividing the genome between two daughter cells.

C. half the number of chromosomes per nucleus, without randomly dividing the genome between two daughter cells.

D. half the number of chromosomes per nucleus, while randomly dividing the genome between two daughter cells.

Passage V (Questions 30–36)

Physiological changes during the human menstrual cycle are affected by levels of sex hormones. The following procedure measured the secretion of estrogens during the menstrual cycle, and also during pregnancy and menopause.

Test subjects were chosen with approximately equal weights and levels of daily activity. Pregnant subjects were tested at the 160th day of the gestational period or at term. Another group of subjects was tested after showing postmenopausal signs and symptoms for at least two months prior to testing. Menstruating subjects were tested either at the onset of menstruation, at the peak of ovulation, or at the luteal maximum. The luteal maximum represents the greatest amount of estrogen secretion during the second half of the menstrual cycle.

During the test period, urine samples were taken every four hours. Urinary levels of five naturally occurring estrogens were measured using the Kober test. The Kober test produces a pink color in the presence of estrogens, including the oxidative product estriol. Estradiol is the most potent estrogen, while estrone is weaker and estriol is the weakest of the three. In Table 1, the results of the procedure are shown, with the value of estrogen levels averaged for each test group.

Estrogen excreted per 24 hours					
Time measurement	Estriol	Estrone	Estradiol	16-Epiestriol	16a-Hydroxy-estrone
Onset of menstruation	7 µg	6 µg	3 µg	*	*
Ovulation peak	28 µg	21 µg	10 µg	*	*
Luteal maximum	23 µg	15 µg	8 µg	*	*
Pregnancy, 160 days	8 mg	0.8 mg	0.3 mg	*	*
Pregnancy, term	31 mg	2.5 mg	0.85 mg	0.80 mg	1.8 mg
Postmenopause	4.3 µg	3.0 µg	0.7 µg	*	*

Table 1

30. Which of the following ovarian cell organelles will show the greatest levels of activity during the secretion of estrogen steroids?

A. Lysosomes
B. Golgi apparatus
C. Plastids
D. Ribosomes

GO ON TO THE NEXT PAGE

31. Which test groups showed the greatest levels of estrogen synthesis and secretion?

    I. Onset of menstruation
   II. Ovulation peak
  III. Pregnancy, 160 days
  IV. Pregnancy, term

    A. I and III
    B. I and IV
    C. II and III
    D. III and IV

32. From Table 1, which variable would prove to be the best marker for the term stage of normal pregnancy, as indicated by the Kober test?

    A. The oxidation of estradiol
    B. The presence of estriol
    C. The presence of 16a-hydroxyestrone
    D. A positive Kober reaction

33. Would estrogen levels in males increase at the onset of puberty?

    A. Yes, because the increased levels of testosterone in the pubertal male are partially converted to estrogens.
    B. Yes, because the increased rate of respiration in pubertal males leads to a decrease in testosterone levels.
    C. No, because estrogen hormones are produced only by abnormal human males.
    D. No, because estrogen hormones do not vary in amount at the onset of puberty in the male.

34. In Table 1, which of the following pairs of subject groups showed the greatest differences in the ratios of estrone to 16-epiestriol levels?

    A. Pregnancy/160 days and postmenopause
    B. Pregnancy/term and pregnancy/160 days
    C. Postmenopause and pregnancy/160 days
    D. Onset of menstruation and postmenopause

35. What change in the ratio of estrone to estradiol is expected to occur as women enter postmenopause, according to the passage?

    A. The ratio increases, because estradiol levels decrease relatively more than estrone levels decrease.
    B. The ratio increases, because estradiol levels decrease while estrone levels are unaffected.
    C. The ratio is unchanged, because both estrogen hormone levels decrease in the postmenopausal period.
    D. The ratio decreases, because estrone levels decrease more than estradiol levels.

36. Researchers further studied estrogen levels in subjects at the luteal minimum of estrogen secretion and at the 210th day of pregnancy. Which findings would NOT indicate a trend similar to that found during the original procedures?

    A. The levels of estriol are greater than the levels of estradiol in both pregnant and luteal minimum groups.
    B. The levels of estradiol are lower than those of estrone in the pregnant group.
    C. The estrone levels are elevated in the pregnant group compared with the luteal minimum group.
    D. The ratio of 16-epiestriol levels between the pregnant and luteal minimum groups is 1:2.

GO ON TO THE NEXT PAGE

Passage VI (Questions 37–42)

The figure illustrates a procedure used in the preparation of organic compounds from alkyl halides. These compounds are useful intermediates for the synthesis of a variety of organic products.

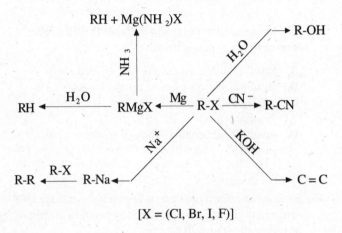

[X = (Cl, Br, I, F)]

Figure 1

37. When alkyl halides react with potassium hydroxide to yield alkene derivatives, the potassium hydroxide acts as:

    A. an acid.
    B. a base.
    C. a proton donor.
    D. a reductant.

38. If one were to substitute heavy water in the last steps of the Grignard reagent, the reaction would lead to the synthesis of:

    A. R-R.
    B. R-OD.
    C. R-D.
    D. R-H.

39. Alkyl halides are not usually prepared by direct halo-genation of alkanes because:

    A. alkanes are not very reactive compounds.
    B. alkanes have low boiling points.
    C. alkanes are desaturated by halogenation.
    D. alkanes do not dissolve in polarized solutions.

40. The synthesis of ethane from ethyl bromide requires the addition of:

    A. Mg and H_2O.
    B. Mg and RCH_2Cl.
    C. Na^+ and RCH_2Cl.
    D. Na^+ and CH_3Br.

41. Alkyl halides are insoluble in water because:

    A. they are hydrophilic.
    B. they are ionic compounds.
    C. they are unable to form hydrogen bonds.
    D. they contain electron-withdrawing groups.

42. Identification of alkyl halides is often based on all of the following physical properties EXCEPT:

    A. boiling point.
    B. density.
    C. spectroscopy.
    D. mass.

GO ON TO THE NEXT PAGE

Passage VII (Questions 43–48)

Carbohydrate absorption is controlled by several factors, including levels of blood glucose. Insulin and glucagon secretion regulates plasma glucose levels in response to blood glucose availability. This is accomplished by a negative feedback control mechanism that regulates cellular metabolism.

In response to high levels of blood glucose, the pancreas secretes insulin into the bloodstream, which acts to increase the availability of plasma glucose to tissues. Glucagon is secreted in response to low levels of blood glucose and acts to decrease plasma glucose availability to tissue cells.

Experiments on laboratory animals illustrate how insulin and glucagon together regulate carbohydrate metabolism. The experimental administration of insulin to laboratory mice has been shown to induce hypoglycemic shock and convulsions. Alternatively, the administration of glucose to animals in hypoglycemic shock causes immediate and dramatic recovery.

Experiment 1

Step 1: A single dose of insulin (50-100 IU/Kg) was administered to an experimental group of laboratory mice. Blood was drawn at 15-minute intervals in order to assay the levels of plasma glucose up until the onset of convulsions.

Step 2: Immediately thereafter, the mice were injected with glucose solution. Glucose administration was continued until convulsions ceased to occur.

Results: Experimental insulin administration caused severe hypoglycemic shock, which was dramatically remedied by the administration of glucose.

Experiment 2 was identical to Experiment 1 except that glucose was administered instead of insulin, thereby inducing hyperglycemia, which was immediately reversed by insulin injection.

43. Which of the following would NOT account for elevated levels of insulin in the blood?

    A. Ingesting a heavy meal
    B. Injecting insulin at bedtime
    C. Arising after an all-night fast
    D. Breaking a fast

44. Which of the following individuals would have the highest levels of glucagon in the bloodstream?

    A. A man running in the last third of a marathon
    B. A pregnant woman after eating breakfast
    C. A bedridden patient two hours after a meal
    D. A child after eating dessert

45. The administration of insulin in Experiment 2 is able to reverse hyperglycemia because:

    A. insulin inhibits glucose uptake by body cells.
    B. insulin enhances glucose uptake by body cells.
    C. glucagon production by the liver is inhibited by insulin.
    D. levels of intracellular glucose are reduced by insulin.

46. From what information can a researcher conclude that insulin and glucagon are produced by two different types of pancreatic islet cells?

    A. Certain islet cells have secretory products similar to those secreted by nervous system cells.
    B. High blood glucose increases the activity of some islet cells, while low blood glucose increases the activity of different islet cell types.
    C. Insulin and glucagon have opposing actions in the body.
    D. Insulin and glucagon have different polypeptide chains.

47. Body cells can respond in vivo to exogenously administered insulin because insulin is a polypeptide that interacts with cells via:

    A. a bilayer membrane that allows simple inward diffusion of insulin.
    B. a bilayer membrane that allows endocytosis of insulin.
    C. cell receptors that are activated in close association with insulin.
    D. cell receptors that degrade insulin on contact.

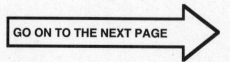
GO ON TO THE NEXT PAGE

48. What happened to the levels of blood glucose in the blood after insulin administration in Experiment 1?

A. Glucose was moved primarily into the liver and not other body tissues.
B. Glucose was moved primarily into the kidneys, as in diabetes insipidus.
C. Glucose was moved into body cells because insulin prevented blood cell degradation of glucose.
D. Glucose was moved into body cells because insulin increased the cells' uptake of glucose.

> Questions 49 through 53 are **NOT** based on a descriptive passage.

49. Bacteriophages are viruses that attack bacteria. They attach to the surface of a bacterium and inject their genetic material into the host. Bacteriophages differ from other living organisms because:

A. they lack the means to replicate inside a host cell.
B. they have only RNA and must utilize a host cell's machinery to generate DNA.
C. they lack the cellular metabolic machinery found in both eukaryotic and prokaryotic organisms.
D. they possess bounding membranes and internal organelles including ribosomes and vacuoles.

50. Consider the reaction below.

$$C_5H_5NH^+$$

$$CH_3CH_2CH_2OH \rightarrow CH_3CH_2CHO$$

Which of the following observations about the infrared spectrum of the reaction mixture would indicate that the reaction shown above occurred?

A. The appearance of a C=O stretch and C–H stretch
B. The appearance of an aliphatic C–H stretch
C. The appearance of an O–H stretch
D. The disappearance of an N–H stretch

51. The process of respiration consists of both inspiration and expiration. Inspiration is:

A. a passive process due to negative pressure in the thoracic cavity.
B. a passive process due to positive pressure in the thoracic cavity.
C. an active process due to negative pressure in the thoracic cavity.
D. an active process due to positive pressure in the thoracic cavity.

52. Sickle cell anemia is a blood disorder due to a point mutation in a single gene. It is inherited as an autosomal recessive trait. A woman is heterozygous for the disorder, having one normal allele on the genome and one allele affected by the point mutation. She most likely has:

A. full-blown sickle cell anemia.
B. sickle cell trait, a carrier disease.
C. no signs or symptoms of the disease.
D. a predominance of sickle-shaped red blood cells.

53. Which of the following is NOT a resonance structure of phenol?

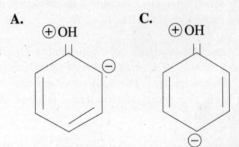

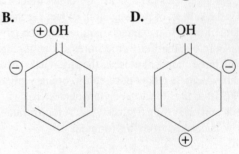

GO ON TO THE NEXT PAGE

Coronary atherosclerosis refers to an accumulation of cholesterol plaques within the coronary arteries and is the principal cause of myocardial infarction ("heart attack"). Coronary atherosclerosis is more common in patients with preexisting high blood pressure and, some authorities believe, in patients who experience high levels of stress. The condition is known to relate closely to the concentration of lipid in the blood.

The bloodstream carries lipids in five different types of lipoprotein particles: (1) chylomicrons, (2) very low-density lipoproteins (VLDL), (3) low-density lipoproteins (LDL), (4) intermediate-density lipoproteins (IDL), and (5) high-density lipoproteins (HDL). All five types of lipoprotein particles share a basic structure. A core of nonpolar lipid is surrounded by a surface coat of phospholipid. At one end the surface phospholipid molecules are polar and therefore soluble in the plasma. At the other end, they are nonpolar and therefore lipid-soluble.

The lipoprotein most often and most strongly associated with coronary atherosclerosis, and hence with the incidence of myocardial infarction, is LDL. The coronary arteries supply the heart muscle itself with blood to meet its metabolic needs. When flow through the coronary arteries is sufficiently compromised by atherosclerosis, a portion of the muscle is damaged or dies for lack of blood supply.

LDL promotes the formation of atherosclerotic plaques in the coronary arteries. HDL particles, on the other hand, tend to prevent atherosclerosis. The lipid imbalance that most commonly leads to coronary atherosclerosis is an excess of LDL relative to HDL.

How derangements in plasma lipoproteins induce atherosclerosis is the subject of investigation. Whatever the precise mechanism, clinical management requires that the physician effectively employ laboratory procedures to identify high-risk states. With three simple blood tests the physician can identify virtually all patients at risk of developing coronary atherosclerosis. The tests are: (1) total serum cholesterol, (2) HDL cholesterol, and (3) fasting triglycerides. A fourth value, LDL cholesterol, is derived from this formula:

LDL cholesterol = (total serum cholesterol – HDL cholesterol)

From 60 percent to 70 percent of serum cholesterol is found in LDL particles, which explains the strong relationship between total serum cholesterol and LDL content. As is shown in Figure 1, the correlation between serum cholesterol and morbidity from atherosclerosis varies with the age group to which the patient belongs.

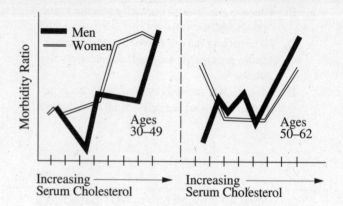

Figure 1

54. High total serum cholesterol puts a patient at risk for myocardial infarction because it reflects:

   A. low blood content of high-density lipoproteins.
   B. low blood content of low-density lipoproteins.
   C. high blood content of high-density lipoproteins.
   D. high blood content of low-density lipoproteins.

55. If an elderly woman with abnormally high levels of LDL has little coronary atherosclerosis, she most likely:

   A. has high levels of HDL, counteracting the effects of the LDL.
   B. follows a diet that is low in cholesterol-containing foods.
   C. has no atherosclerosis in arteries outside the heart.
   D. has failed to undergo a complete diagnostic screening for blood lipid status.

56. Coronary atherosclerosis constitutes a medical problem because it threatens to:

   A. render the heart less sensitive to stress.
   B. produce imbalance in the patient's blood lipid profile.
   C. compromise the heart muscle's oxygen supply.
   D. subject the patient to high blood pressure.

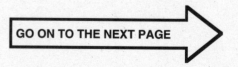

GO ON TO THE NEXT PAGE

57. Coronary atherosclerosis is virtually unknown among peoples living in non-industrialized nations. This indicates that in comparison with industrialized populations these peoples probably have:

A. a lower incidence of heart attack.
B. a lower incidence of hypertension.
C. higher levels of VLDL.
D. higher levels of IDL.

58. If coronary atherosclerosis produces myocardial infarction, what is the status of the affected heart muscle?

A. High pH
B. Low pH
C. High O_2 concentration
D. Low CO_2 concentration

Passage IX (Questions 59–65)

In studying the effect of molecular substituents on the acidity of carboxylic acids, researchers have compared equilibrium reactions for the deprotonation of a number of dicarboxylic acids. A standard reaction for comparison purposes is the deprotonation of malonic acid.

$$HOOCCH_2COOH \rightarrow HOOCCH_2COO^- + H^+$$

Reaction I

The equilibrium rate constant for Reaction I is symbolized as K_1. The anion in Reaction I can be further deprotonated; the equilibrium constant for this reaction is symbolized as K_2, a value substantially lower than the original K_1.

$$HOOCCH_2COO^- \rightarrow {}^-OOCCH_2COO^- + H^+$$

Reaction II

The constants K_1 and K_2 are determined according to the following equations:

$$K_1 = \frac{\left[HOOCCH_2COO^-\right]\left[H^+\right]}{\left[HOOCCH_2COOH\right]} \quad K_2 = \frac{\left[{}^-OOCCH_2COO^-\right]\left[H^+\right]}{\left[HOOCCH_2COO^-\right]}$$

The ratios above are determined under equilibrium conditions and do not apply to non-equilibrium conditions.

The table below lists the values of K_1 and K_2 for several dicarboxylic acids.

Compound	Formula	K_1	K_2
Oxalic Acid	HOOC—COOH	5400×10^{-5}	5.2×10^{-5}
Malonic Acid	$HOOCCH_2COOH$	140×10^{-5}	0.2×10^{-5}
Succinic Acid	$HOOC(CH_2)_2COOH$	64×10^{-5}	0.23×10^{-5}
Maleic Acid	HOOCCH=CHCOOH	1000×10^{-5}	0.055×10^{-5}
Fumaric Acid	HOOCCH=CHCOOH	96×10^{-5}	4.1×10^{-5}

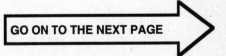

GO ON TO THE NEXT PAGE

Note: The structures of fumaric and maleic acid are shown below:

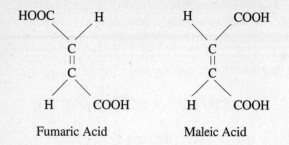

Fumaric Acid   Maleic Acid

59. In studying the passage, one could estimate a dicarboxylic acid's K_1 value by determining:

   A. its concentration in a non-equilibrium mixture.
   B. its stability in anion form.
   C. its tendency to undergo decarboxylation.
   D. its crystallization structure.

60. Glutaric acid is a dicarboxylic acid with formula $HOOC(CH_2)_3COOH$. This acid is most likely to have a K_1 constant closest in value to which substance listed in the table?

   A. Fumaric acid
   B. Maleic acid
   C. Succinic acid
   D. Oxalic acid

61. If equal concentrations of succinic acid, malonic acid, and maleic acid were heated in a weakly basic solution, which of the following products would be in the greatest concentration at equilibrium?

   A. $HOOCCH_2COO^-$
   B. $HOOC(CH_2)_2COO^-$
   C. *trans*-$HOOCCH=CHCOOH$
   D. $HOOC-COOH$

62. In applying the information in the passage, it would be difficult to estimate K_1 for a molecule with the formula $HOOCCH_2NHCOOH$ because:

   A. its anion stability is not directly comparable to that of succinic acid.
   B. it cannot exist in the deprotonated form.
   C. it must form an insoluble compound.
   D. it represents an unstable compound.

63. In an aqueous mixture of maleic and fumaric acid, the equilibrium proportions can best be determined by which method?

   A. Radioactive tagging of the corresponding alkene
   B. Hydration of the anion solution
   C. Acidification of the solution
   D. Nuclear magnetic resonance spectroscopy of the equilibrium solution

64. The value of K_1 of the dicarboxylic compound glutamic acid is substantially lower than the K_1 of glutaric acid because:

   A. glutamate is readily convertible into a nonpolar Zwitterion.
   B. glutamate's deprotonated form is less stable than the glutarate anion.
   C. glutamate is an amino acid.
   D. glutamic acid is a stronger acid than glutaric acid.

65. One can most reasonably estimate the value of K_2 for acetic acid (CH_3COOH) to be:

   A. higher than K_1 for acetic acid.
   B. higher than K_2 for maleic acid.
   C. lower than K_2 for oxalic acid.
   D. less than zero.

GO ON TO THE NEXT PAGE

Bacillus subtilis is a gram-positive bacterium that reproduces itself through replication of a double-stranded chromosome. Reproduction does not require the formation of gametes. The haploid cells of *B. subtilis* undergo asexual division in which the haploid number is preserved and two daughter cells are formed from one parent. *B. subtilis* does not form a diploid state, and does not undergo a reduction division. In studying *B. subtilis* scientists have also studied bacteriophage SP8, a virus that infects *B. subtilis*. Of particular interest is that the virus performs transcription from a single strand of intact double-stranded viral DNA using host cell enzymatic machinery.

Experiment 1

To determine the role of each DNA strand in transcription, researchers denatured the viral DNA and hybridized the separated strands, termed Light and Heavy, to tritiated RNA isolated from SP8-infected *B. subtilis*. The density of the separated strands was determined, and the hybridized DNA-RNA strands were analyzed in the presence of RNAse, a hydrolytic enzyme. The graphs in Figure 1 and Figure 2 summarize the results obtained for both Light and Heavy strands of viral DNA.

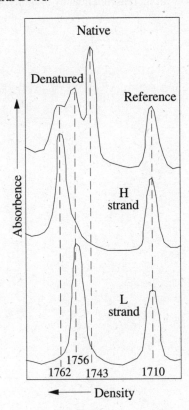

Figure 1

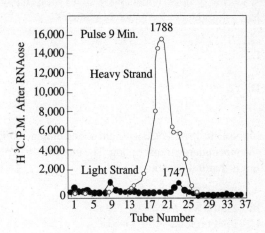

Figure 2

Experiment 2

SP8-infected *B. subtilis*, carrying the viral DNA, was induced to undergo division, and the viral DNA Light strand of one daughter cell was extensively mutated. The other daughter's viral DNA Light strand was unaffected. There were no phenotypic differences between the daughter cells, including reproduction rates.

Experiment 3

SP8-infected *B. subtilis* was again induced to undergo division. The Light strand of viral DNA of one daughter cell was extensively mutated, and the Heavy strand of viral DNA of the second daughter was also mutated. The two daughter cells were induced to undergo a second round of division. Only the daughter cell with the mutated viral DNA Light strand produced offspring. The two Light strand mutants were again induced to replicate and successfully produced offspring.

66. If a segment of the denatured viral DNA strand had a base sequence ATAA, what would have been the complementary RNA sequence?

   A. GTGG
   B. TATT
   C. UAUU
   D. TUTT

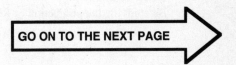

GO ON TO THE NEXT PAGE

67. At the end of Experiment 3, how many offspring reproduced through the formation of gametes?

- **A.** 0
- **B.** 2
- **C.** 4
- **D.** 12

68. Suppose the lower-density Light strand mutant in Figure 1 cannot undergo transcription. The most likely explanation is that it does not:

- **A.** bind DNA.
- **B.** bind RNA.
- **C.** bind protein.
- **D.** replicate.

69. Mutated viral DNA Light strand produces no abnormal phenotypic changes, which is most likely due to the fact that the viral DNA Light strand:

- **A.** does not undergo translation.
- **B.** does not undergo replication.
- **C.** is contained in the nucleus.
- **D.** is able to undergo translation.

70. On what finding could one base the conclusion that the viral DNA Heavy strand normally produces transcribed mRNA, whereas the viral DNA Light strand does not?

- **A.** Neither the Heavy strand nor the Light strand of viral DNA can excise point mutations.
- **B.** Neither the Heavy strand nor the Light strand of viral DNA hybridizes with labeled RNA.
- **C.** Only mutated viral DNA Heavy strands exist in the natural setting.
- **D.** Only the mutated viral DNA Heavy strand produces phenotypic changes.

71. How can one conclude that mutations of the viral DNA Light strand do not affect phenotypic expression in the host?

- **A.** By locating the mutation on the host DNA
- **B.** By comparing Light strand mutants with Heavy strand mutants
- **C.** By comparing the mutant phenotype with the unmutated form
- **D.** By studying the production of RNA polymerase

72. By studying Figures 1 and 2, a scientist decided that the normal bacteriophage SP8 DNA consists of a double-stranded chromosome. For this conclusion to be true, which of the following assumptions must be correct?

- **A.** Hybridization of DNA with RNA involves the formation of covalent bonds.
- **B.** Radio-labeling affects the size of the RNA-DNA hybrid produced.
- **C.** Mutation does not lead to changes in DNA sequence.
- **D.** Denaturation breaks apart the double helix without hydrolyzing covalently attached base pairs.

73. For bacteriophage SP8, if the mutated Heavy strand codes for a protein that destroys DNA polymerases while the Light strand does not, then the mutant will:

- **A.** show increased production of DNA.
- **B.** show decreased evolutionary "fitness" compared with the Light strand mutant.
- **C.** show increased evolutionary "fitness" compared with the normal virus.
- **D.** show an increased tendency to undergo meiosis.

Questions 74 through 77 are **NOT** based on a descriptive passage.

74. Which of the following processes does NOT occur on the ribosomes during protein synthesis?

   A. Translation of mRNA
   B. Peptide bond formation
   C. Attachment of tRNA anticodons to mRNA codons
   D. Attachment of mRNA anticodons to tRNA codons

75. During embryonic gastrulation, invagination occurs as a result of which of the following processes?

   A. Release of a hormone
   B. Migration of cells
   C. Reproduction of cells
   D. Asymmetric division of cells

76. Surgically implanted pacemakers are frequently used in the treatment of heart disease. Which of the following normal heart structures carries out the same function as a pacemaker?

   A. The bundle of His
   B. The atrio-ventricular node
   C. The sino-atrial node
   D. The sino-ventricular node

77. The hormone that most directly stimulates the formation of sperm in the testes is which of the following?

   A. Estrogen
   B. Testosterone
   C. Luteinizing hormone
   D. Follicle-stimulating hormone

STOP
IF YOU FINISH BEFORE TIME IS CALLED, YOU MAY CHECK YOUR WORK ON THIS TEST ONLY. DO NOT TURN TO ANY OTHER TEST IN THIS BOOK.

DIAGNOSTIC TEST ANSWERS

Section 1 Verbal Reasoning		Section 2 Physical Sciences		Section 3 Biological Sciences	
1. C	34. B	1. B	40. C	1. B	40. A
2. A	35. B	2. A	41. C	2. A	41. C
3. D	36. C	3. C	42. A	3. D	42. D
4. B	37. B	4. D	43. B	4. C	43. C
5. B	38. C	5. D	44. D	5. C	44. A
6. A	39. B	6. B	45. C	6. A	45. B
7. A	40. B	7. B	46. D	7. C	46. B
8. D	41. D	8. D	47. B	8. A	47. C
9. D	42. A	9. A	48. D	9. B	48. D
10. B	43. C	10. B	49. A	10. A	49. C
11. B	44. C	11. B	50. B	11. D	50. A
12. D	45. B	12. B	51. B	12. D	51. C
13. A	46. B	13. C	52. B	13. B	52. B
14. C	47. B	14. B	53. B	14. C	53. D
15. B	48. D	15. C	54. C	15. B	54. D
16. C	49. B	16. B	55. C	16. C	55. A
17. A	50. D	17. B	56. B	17. A	56. C
18. C	51. B	18. D	57. D	18. A	57. A
19. B	52. C	19. A	58. D	19. C	58. B
20. B	53. A	20. B	59. B	20. C	59. B
21. D	54. A	21. C	60. A	21. D	60. C
22. A	55. D	22. B	61. D	22. B	61. A
23. B	56. B	23. C	62. A	23. D	62. A
24. D	57. C	24. C	63. D	24. C	63. D
25. A	58. B	25. C	64. B	25. C	64. B
26. C	59. A	26. C	65. C	26. D	65. C
27. B	60. B	27. B	66. A	27. B	66. C
28. A	61. D	28. A	67. D	28. A	67. A
29. C	62. B	29. A	68. D	29. B	68. B
30. B	63. A	30. C	69. A	30. B	69. A
31. C	64. A	31. D	70. A	31. D	70. D
32. A	65. C	32. D	71. C	32. C	71. C
33. C		33. B	72. B	33. A	72. D
		34. C	73. C	34. B	73. B
		35. A	74. A	35. A	74. D
		36. B	75. B	36. D	75. B
		37. C	76. C	37. B	76. C
		38. B	77. B	38. C	77. B
		39. D		39. A	

SCORE CONVERSION CHART

Verbal Reasoning

Total Correct	Scaled Score
65	15
64	14
62–63	13
60–61	12
58–59	11
55–57	10
50–54	9
45–49	8
39–44	7
33–38	6
27–32	5
22–26	4
17–21	3
11–16	2
0–10	1

Physical Sciences

Total Correct	Scaled Score
76–77	15
73–75	14
69–72	13
63–68	12
57–62	11
51–56	10
46–50	9
39–45	8
34–38	7
28–33	6
23–27	5
18–22	4
13–17	3
8–12	2
0–7	1

Biological Sciences

Total Correct	Scaled Score
76–77	15
74–75	14
70–73	13
67–69	12
63–66	11
58–62	10
53–57	9
46–52	8
40–45	7
34–39	6
28–33	5
24–27	4
20–23	3
15–19	2
0–14	1

PART III

MCAT DIAGNOSTIC TEST ANSWERS: EXPLANATIONS

Passage I (Questions 1–7)

1. According to the passage, Einstein's theory of relativity states that:

   A. time is absolute for all objects traveling at or near the speed of light.
   B. the speed of light varies, depending on the observer's frame of reference.
   C. time varies for different frames of reference, but the speed of light does not.
   D. time is absolute, but space is not.

1. **C is correct.** In paragraph 2 the author tells you that, in the Newtonian world time is independent of reference. In paragraph 3, she tells you that Einstein's theory "put an end to the concept of absolute time. . . . [Each] frame of reference carries its own system of time." The very next sentence tells you that Einstein's theory "recognizes only one absolute parameter: the speed of light. That is constant in all frames of reference. . . ."

   The wrong answer choices: Choices A, B, and D all contradict the passage. The author states that Einstein did *not* consider time to be absolute and that he did consider the speed of light to be absolute.

2. The author suggests that the theory of relativity:

    A. is inconsistent with Newtonian views of the universe.
    B. contradicts the Michelson-Morley experiment.
    C. is valid only for two observers in the same frame of reference.
    D. cannot be proven right or wrong.

2. **A** is correct. In the first sentence of the second paragraph, you're told that "Einstein's theory of relativity . . . required that humanity *abandon* the Newtonian notion. . . ." In other words, relativity can't stand side by side with Newtonian physics. The two perspectives are mutually inconsistent.

The wrong answer choices: Choices B and C take the author's words and distort their meaning. The author does refer to the Michelson-Morley experiment, but she never even hints that Einstein's theory is at odds with it. At the end of paragraph 3, she writes that Einstein's theory "constitutes a recognition of the Michelson-Morley findings." The author also cites illustrations involving two observers, and she refers to the phrase "frame of reference." She nowhere suggests, however, that Einstein's theory is valid only for two observers in the same frame of reference. Choice D is wild.

3. The author indicates that under the relativity theory, unlike earlier theories:

    A. mass and energy are conserved only in reactions taking place on Earth.
    B. all mass has the inherent ability to travel faster than light.
    C. neither mass nor energy can ever be converted or destroyed.
    D. energy may be transformed to mass, and mass may be transformed to energy.

3. **D** is correct. In paragraph 5, the author tells you that one of Einstein's theorems means that "all mass is energy, that all energy is mass, and that the two are interconvertible." This question tests your ability to see that choice D makes, more or less, the same statement in different words. To say that mass and energy are *interconvertible* is to say that energy may be transformed to mass and that mass may be transformed to energy.

The wrong answer choices: Choice A takes the author's words and distorts their meaning. The author notes that at *Earthly velocities* the interconvertibility of mass and energy are not noticeable. This has nothing to do with any notion that mass is conserved only in reactions taking place on Earth. Choice B is contrary to the passage. You're told that according to Einstein, nothing can exceed the speed of light. Choice C is also contrary to the passage. Einstein's theory provides that mass and energy *are* interconvertible.

4. The fact that most motion we deal with day to day involves speeds far less than that of light means that:

   A. two observers cannot appreciate the fact that their frames of reference may differ.
   B. we are not aware that moving objects experience changes in mass.
   C. we cannot view motion according to the Newtonian model.
   D. we do not perceive any difference between the parameters of space and time.

4. **B** is correct. According to paragraph 5, the interconvertibility of mass and energy are unnoticeable at "Earthly velocities," meaning velocities far below the speed of light. Only as objects attain speeds approaching that of light do changes in their mass become apparent. At velocities far below the speed of light, you're told, the effect is not detectable.

The wrong answer choices: Choices A and D are more or less doubletalk. They take the author's words and distort their meaning beyond recognition. The author alludes to frames of reference, to observers, and to space and time. *Nowhere* does she make statements akin to the one set forth in choice A. Choice C is wholly unwarranted. We are told in paragraph 5 that at speeds less than the speed of light, motion does not appear to follow *Einstein's* theory.

5. According to the passage, the equation $E = mc^2$ represents:

   A. a new manner of describing a longstanding physical law.
   B. a highly innovative view of the relationship between two well-known parameters.
   C. an alternative formulation of the Michelson-Morley hypothesis.
   D. a direct outgrowth of Newtonian physics.

5. **B** is correct. At the beginning of paragraph 5, the author describes Einstein's "revolutionary discovery" that mass and energy are equivalent. This discovery, you're told, is tied in with the equation $E = mc^2$. In order to answer this question, you need only recognize that (1) "highly innovative view" is intended to mean, more or less, the same thing as "revolutionary discovery," and (2) mass and energy are well-known parameters.

6. According to Einstein, two observers will agree on the time at which a single event occurs only if:

   A. they are in the same frame of reference.
   B. they apply Newtonian laws of motion.
   C. they refer to clocks of varying mass.
   D. they move in opposite directions at or near the speed of light.

6. **A** is correct. In paragraph 3, you're told that "a frame of reference carries its own system of time." Hence, two observers will agree on the time at which an event occurs only if they are in the *same* frame of reference.

The wrong answer choices: Choices B, C, and D borrow the author's words and phrases and distort their meaning. The author refers, of course, to Newtonian laws of motion, to clocks, to mass, to directions, and to the speed of light. Nowhere, however, does she make any statements remotely resembling the ones set forth in choices B, C, and D.

7. Which of the following findings would weaken the theory of relativity as it is described in the passage?

   I. Certain subatomic particles and waves travel at speeds that exceed the speed of light.
   II. The speed of sound is dependent on the medium in which it travels.
   III. No known Earthly object has ever achieved a speed equal to that of light.

   A. I only
   B. III only
   C. I and II only
   D. I, II, and III

7. **A** is correct. The question requires simple logic. According to the theory of relativity, you're told, nothing can exceed the speed of light. Option I suggests that some particles and waves do exceed the speed of light. If that proposition were true, it would be inconsistent with the theory of relativity and would thus weaken it considerably. Option III is fully consistent with the theory, and option II is irrelevant to it.

8. The author probably compares the situations of a six-month-old and six-year-old taken to the theater in order to demonstrate that:

    A. fully socialized adults must take responsibility for less socialized children.
    B. children who are exposed to music and art will experience faster maturation.
    C. older children have greater appreciation for culture than do younger children.
    D. an older child is likely to be more socialized than a younger child.

8. **D** is correct. In paragraph 1, the author makes a general point: "In the process of socialization, the child learns to respect the rights and property of others." The very next sentence tells you what socialization *is*. The socialized child is able to "conform behavior to the circumstances that surround him or her at any given time." In order to answer this question, you have to see that the illustration involving the theater supports the point that an older child is better able than a younger child to "conform behavior to the circumstances." In other words, the author intends to demonstrate that an older child is better socialized than a younger child.

    The wrong answer choices: Choice A is wrong because it is irrelevant to the main thrust of the paragraph and the passage. Choices B and C are also wrong because they bear no connection to the author's points.

9. Which of the following statements represents the most sensible use of the information in the passage?

    A. Children could begin to study foreign language at an early age.
    B. Schoolteachers could use the information to improve training of reading-disabled children.
    C. Parents might use the information to promote more productive interactions among their several children.
    D. Sociologists might use the information to expand their understanding of socialization.

9. **D** is correct. The passage offers a new approach to the understanding of socialization. You're supposed to figure out, therefore, that a sociologist might use the information to gain a better understanding of socialization.

    The wrong answer choices: Choices A and C are wrong because they incorporate the author's words but distort his meaning. The author refers to language, interactions, and parents but never makes points relevant to the matters described in choices A or C. Choice B is wrong because it is far removed from the author's discussions.

10. A social psychologist conducted a study in which one hundred eight-year-olds were observed knocking on a door to call on a playmate. When each child was asked by a parent whom he wished to see, 90 percent identified the playmate by name. Given the discussion in the passage, it is most reasonable to conclude that:

A. Some eight-year-olds are far more independent of their parents than others.
B. Most eight-year-olds are better able to identify a person by name than by his relationship to others.
C. Most eight-year-olds have no concern for the relationship between another child and that child's parent.
D. Most eight-year-olds think of themselves as fully independent beings, not as the children of their parents.

11. By the age of six months, most children have developed the ability to wave "bye-bye" to departing persons. Professor Speier would most likely view this development as:

A. unrelated to the process of socialization.
B. the achievement of a specific interactional ability.
C. a crucial stage in the child's ability to process information.
D. a reflection of the child's ability to cope with separations and absence.

10. B is correct. The author takes trouble to point out that an eight-year-old, when speaking to a playmate's parent, has the ability to identify a playmate as "your son." Bearing in mind that this is important to the author's discussion, you should recognize that B is the intended answer. B indicates that eight-year-olds have *not* developed the ability to which the author refers.

The wrong answer choices: Choice A sounds reasonable and "nice," but it has nothing to do with the author's points. Choice C is an extreme ("*no* concern"). An answer choice is seldom correct if it talks in absolutes. Choice D is far removed from the author's discussion.

11. B is correct. Speier's main point is basically this: Socialization is a process in which children develop their ability to *interact*. In order to answer this question, you should keep that point in mind and find the choice that most closely corresponds to it. That's why B is right.

The wrong answer choices: Choice A is wrong because it is contrary to the passage's central purpose and Speier's viewpoints. Choice C sounds sensible, but it is unrelated to the points made in the passage. Choice D borrows the words "separation" and "absence" from paragraph 2, but thoroughly distorts the author's meaning. The author noted only that the ability to accept temporary absence and separation marked developmental progress. There is nothing in the passage to suggest that a child's ability to wave goodbye has bearing on her ability to accept separation or absence.

12. Speier views the situation involving the child who called at his playmate's home (lines 46–53) as demonstrating that:

A. socialization and interaction are entirely separate developmental processes.
B. children are better able to interact with other children than with adults.
C. children do not understand the role they themselves play in interaction.
D. the ability to interact competently with others involves a number of separate interactional abilities.

13. Matthew Speier's views are relevant to sociology because they:

A. suggest a new conceptual framework within which to view the socialization process.
B. name discrete developmental stages by which children can be evaluated.
C. classify all forms of interaction between children and adults.
D. confirm all aspects of the classical view of socialization.

12. **D** is correct. The sixth paragraph specifically describes two interactional abilities. The words "first" and "second" tell you that. Furthermore, choice D reflects Speier's thesis: that socialization represents increased ability to *interact*.

The wrong answer choices: Choice A is wrong because it directly contradicts Speier's thesis. Speier believes that socialization is intimately involved with interaction. Choice B is irrelevant to the passage and the question. Choice C is far removed from the author's discussion.

13. **A** is correct. The question requires that you understand, in summary, the significance of Matthew Speier's point of view as it is described in the passage. In paragraph 2, the author describes classical views of socialization. In paragraph 3, the author tells you that "Matthew Speier . . . feels that socialization might be understood in other terms." The author then goes on to describe Speier's views, which amount to a new approach to socialization. That's why A is right.

The wrong answer choices: Choice B is wrong because you are not told that Speier has attached any names to developmental stages. Furthermore, the notion of "discrete stages" is associated with classical views, not Speier's. Choices C and D are extremes. The word "all" should make you wary of C and D.

14. The main point of the passage is that:

   A. interaction is only one of many competencies that create a fully socialized human being.
   B. children of similar age vary sharply in their development because of diverse interactional abilities.
   C. it may be possible to understand the socialization process in terms of interactional development.
   D. adults should be understanding of children's natural interactional disabilities.

15. As used in the passage, the phrase "referent terms" means:

   A. expressions with which people of diverse backgrounds are likely to be familiar.
   B. words that enable a listener to relate a subject to himself.
   C. phrases that allow a speaker to describe diverse relationships in a single communication.
   D. sentences that do not employ proper names.

14. C is correct. The question requires that you understand the author's central purpose and distinguish it from ancillary points he may make. The passage points out, primarily, that socialization might be viewed in terms of interaction.

   The wrong answer choices: Choice A is wrong because it represents a view that the author *never* expresses. Choices B and D are appealing because they sound sensible and "nice." Unfortunately, they have nothing whatsoever to do with the passage.

15. B is correct. In the last paragraph, the author implicitly explains the meaning of referent terms. You're told that the phrase "your son" was a referent term because it allowed the mother to refer the child's statement *to herself.* Hence, you're supposed to figure out that a referent term is one that allows a listener to relate a subject to himself.

   The wrong answer choices: Choices A, C, and D are wild and irrelevant.

16. Why are geologists unable to study events that occurred between the Mesozoic and Cenozoic era?

    A. The deposition of rock was not a continuous phenomenon.

    B. There was no life during that period.

    C. The rocks provide no record of that interval.

    D. There are no classes intermediate between reptiles and mammals.

16. C is correct. In the last paragraph, you're told that "the record has been broken," which is why events falling between the Mesozoic and Cenozoic era are "lost to us." The rocks offer us no record of that period. That's why C is right.

The wrong answer choices: Choice A is wrong because it directly contradicts the first line of paragraph 5. Choice B represents an unwarranted conclusion. Nothing in the passage encourages the reader to conclude that the interval between the Mesozoic and Cenozoic era was lifeless. Choice D is contrary to a statement made in paragraph 5 where the author writes, "The Earth was *not* one day populated with reptiles and on the next populated with large mammals." The author thus implies that there *were* life forms intermediate between reptiles and mammals.

17. Which of the following is common to Paleozoic and Proterozoic life?

    A. Dependence on proximity to water.

    B. Increased sophistication over Mesozoic organisms.

    C. Presence of small mammals.

    D. Colonization of land masses.

17. A is correct. Paragraph 3 tells you that Proterozoic life was absolutely confined to the water. Paragraph 4 tells you that Paleozoic life remained close to the sea.

The wrong answer choices: Choice B is wrong because you're told in paragraph 2 that the Mesozoic period *came after* the Proterozoic and Paleozoic eras. Choices C and D are wrong because they contradict the passage. You're told that the land masses were devoid of life in both Proterozoic and Paleozoic eras. Small mammals, the author says, appeared in the late but not even the *early Mesozoic* era. Hence, there were *no* mammals during the Proterozoic era.

18. The passage suggests that the appearance of rock formations in distinctly identifiable layers means that:

   A. most rock deposits fail to supply meaningful information concerning the evolution of life.
   B. evolution was not as gradual a process as is often believed.
   C. widespread environmental changes prevented some deposits from being preserved.
   D. all life also developed according to discrete stages and periods.

19. Imagine that a newly discovered rock deposit is explored and that geologists are studying fossils contained in the Cenozoic layer. From information contained in the passage, the geologists would be LEAST likely to discover:

   A. prominence of mammalian life forms.
   B. preponderance of great reptilian organisms.
   C. evidence of life expanding beyond bodies of water and shorelines.
   D. large variety of fish and marine organisms.

18. **C** is correct. Paragraph 5 tells you that "widespread changes . . . caused much deposition to be lost. . . ." Choice C makes, more or less, the same statement.

The wrong answer choices: Choice A is wrong because it contradicts the passage. The author tells you that fossil rock formations *do* provide a valuable record of Earthly life. Choices B and D represent statements that are wholly unwarranted and removed from the passage.

19. **B** is correct. Paragraph 4 associates large reptiles with the *Mesozoic* period, not with the Cenozoic period. Moreover, paragraph 5 implies that in the Cenozoic era, there had been "a near-complete disappearance" of the reptiles.

The wrong answer choices: A, C, and D all make statements that are consistent with the author's description of the Cenozoic era. The author tells you that mammals were prominent in the Cenozoic period. He also says that land was colonized in the Mesozoic period, which *preceded* the Cenozoic. The passage implies that there were a large variety of life forms as early as the Proterozoic period. That means that life was quite varied in the Cenozoic period as well.

20. If an early Paleozoic rock deposit revealed fossils of small mammals, this discovery would weaken which of the following assertions made in the passage?

    I. The age of the mammals was a part of the Cenozoic era.

   II. Mammalian life first appeared in the late Mesozoic era.

  III. Archeozoic life was confined entirely to the water.

  A. I only
  B. II only
  C. I and III only
  D. II and III only

20. B is correct. In paragraph 4, you're told that mammalian life first appeared in the late part of the Mesozoic era. In paragraph 2, you learn that the Mesozoic came *after* the Paleozoic. If mammalian fossils were found in early Paleozoic rocks, it could not be true that mammals *first* appeared in the Mesozoic period. Option I could still be true, since "the age of mammals" refers to their proliferation and development, not their first appearance. Since the Archeozoic era preceded the Paleozoic, option III would be unaffected.

21. According to the passage, the great reptiles were destroyed by a sudden cataclysm with widespread effects across the Earth. On what evidence is this assertion based?

  A. Most mammals living during the Paleozoic period were small.
  B. No reptiles exist on the Earth today.
  C. Some rock deposits present a record of the period between the Mesozoic and Cenozoic in which mammals and reptiles actively competed.
  D. The life forms of the Mesozoic and Cenozoic are dramatically different.

21. D is correct. In paragraph 5, the author writes of the difference between the Mesozoic and Cenozoic records: "The fact that the record should reveal . . . a *near-complete disappearance of an older genus and highly evolved organisms of a new and different one* suggests that the entire Earth must have experienced some tremendous cataclysm..."

The wrong answer choices: Choices A and C contradict the passage. You're told that mammals did not appear until the late *Mesozoic* era. You're also told that there is *no record* of the period between the Mesozoic and Cenozoic eras. Choice B is wild and false.

22. If the fossilized remains of an unknown species were found in a Proterozoic rock deposit, one might most reasonably conclude that the organism:

A. lived in the water.
B. lived among rock.
C. had no need for oxygen.
D. became extinct because of a cataclysmic event.

22. A is correct. You learn in paragraph 3 that all Proterozoic life was confined to water. It's as simple as that.

The wrong answer choices: Choices B and D borrow words and phrases from the passage but distort the author's meaning. The author refers to small *mammals* scampering among the rocks. Elsewhere, he refers to cataclysmic events, but the reference has nothing to do with the extinction of Proterozoic life forms. Choice C is wild and ridiculous.

23. Which of the following observations would best support the hypothesis that reptiles evolved directly from amphibians?

A. Early amphibians and reptiles differed dramatically from one another in their physiology and behavior.
B. Fossil remains of the earliest reptiles resemble those of the amphibians.
C. Most reptiles were extinct before the first amphibians appeared.
D. Both amphibians and reptiles are represented today by a relatively few species.

23. B is correct. In paragraph 5, the author refers to the evolution of life as a "gradual blending and melding of older life forms into newer ones." In order to answer the question you must reason, simply, that when one genus evolves directly from another, the two genuses should resemble each other. That's why B is right.

The wrong answer choices: Choice A is wrong because it contradicts the reasoning just described. Choice C is wrong for this reason: If amphibians were extinct before reptiles arose, it would be *impossible* for reptiles to arise from amphibians. Choice D is wild and irrelevant.

24. Among the following, the finding that fossilized whale remains first appear after the great reptiles have disappeared would LEAST support the conclusion that:

A. whales and reptiles require different environments for their survival.
B. whales evolved directly from early mammals.
C. whales evolved from early Cenozoic aquatic animals.
D. whales and great reptiles co-existed during the Mesozoic era.

24. D is correct. If whales and reptile fossils show marked separation in time, then one should be least inclined to conclude that whales and reptiles co-existed. Rather, one should tentatively conclude, perhaps, that they did *not* co-exist.

The wrong answer choices: Choice A is irrelevant. It has nothing to do with time. Choices B and C are perfectly consistent with the finding described in the question.

Passage IV (Questions 25–30)

25. The passage suggests that the amount of child support that is owed but not paid each year:

    A. will probably increase in spite of congressional action.

    B. is likely to decrease if the adequacy gap is eliminated.

    C. may experience a decrease in response to congressional action.

    D. will remain relatively constant across state lines.

25. **A** is correct. In paragraph 2, you're told about the compliance gap, which refers to the amount of child support that is owed but not paid. You're told that "regardless" of congressional action, the compliance gap will likely increase.

The wrong answer choices: Choices B and C contradict the author's statements. The author says that the compliance gap will increase regardless of congressional action. Choice D is irrelevant. The author says nothing about the relative size of the compliance gap among the several states.

26. The author indicates that Congress took action in the area of child support partially in order to:

    A. encourage both custodial and noncustodial parents to assume responsibility for their children's support.

    B. address the fact that noncustodial parents were not complying with support orders.

    C. correct the unfairness produced by state judges who apply diverse criteria in setting awards.

    D. see that all noncustodial parents paid child support in accordance with a single flat rate formula.

26. **C** is correct. In paragraph 3, the author indicates that, with respect to the establishment of child support awards, state judges are not consistent with one another. The author alludes to the problem in connection with his description of the new federal program and its purpose.

The wrong answer choices: Choices A and B sound sensible and "nice," but they're irrelevant to the question. The author simply does not indicate that Congress intended its new program specifically to encourage support from both parents, nor to address the compliance problem. Choice D is wrong because it contradicts the passage. The author explains that the federal system will allow states to *choose between* the flat rate model and the income shares model.

27. According to the passage, one aim of the income shares approach to child support is to:

    A. put custodial and noncustodial parents in identical economic positions.
    B. prevent divorce from interfering with the child's economic life.
    C. place the child with the parent best able to provide for him.
    D. ease the economic burden that divorce places on custodial parents.

27. **B** is correct. The answer essentially restates the first sentence of paragraph 5: ". . . the income shares model embodies the idea that each child should receive [the income she would have received] had the parents not separated." It's as simple as that.

The wrong answer choices: Choice A is extreme. You should be suspicious of choices that pivot on words like "all," "always," "perfect," "total," "complete," "never," "impossible," and "identical." Choice C seems sensible and sweet. Unfortunately, it has nothing to do with the question or the passage. Choice D represents an unwarranted statement. You simply are *not* told that the income shares model was designed to produce fairness for parents.

28. Given the discussion set forth in the passage, one might justifiably conclude that child support awards will:

    A. begin to reflect more objective rather than subjective criteria.
    B. experience a gradual decline as the new federal law operates.
    C. be oriented less toward the needs of the child and more toward the needs of parents.
    D. cease to become an important component of separation and divorce proceedings.

28. **A** is correct. The question tests your ability to understand paragraph 3. The federal law is designed to address this problem: Child support awards are the product of individual judges acting pursuant to their own standards. Awards are *sub*jective. The new law is designed to make them more *ob*jective.

The wrong answer choices: Choices B and C cannot be deduced from the passage. Choice D, while "nice," cannot be deduced either.

29. Before the new federal law took effect, the passage indicates, a judge's role in setting child support awards might best be described as:

    I. determinative.
    II. relatively insignificant.
    III. largely unregulated.

    A. I only
    B. II only
    C. I and III only
    D. I, II, and III

29. **C** is correct. Paragraphs 1 and 3 tell you that (1) child support awards are issued by state judges and (2) the judges don't have meaningful rules or criteria on which to operate. The judges are totally responsible for setting awards, but they have few rules from which to work. That's why options I and III represent true statements. Option II is contrary to what you're told. The judge's role is all-important.

30. The passage indicates that similarly situated parents in different states may continue to experience different treatment because:

    I. judges are unlikely to abandon their own personal opinions in favor of legal criteria.

   II. separate states may adopt divergent criteria for setting support awards.

  III. the flat rate model does not take account of the custodial parent's income.

  A. I only
  B. II only
  C. I and III only
  D. I, II, and III

30. B is correct. In order to answer the question, you have to realize that the phrase "divergent criteria for setting support awards" refers to the fact that states will choose between the flat rate and income shares models, as described in paragraphs 4 and 5. If one state should choose the flat rate model and another the income shares approach, then the two would be adopting "divergent criteria." Option I is wild and unjustified. Option III represents a true statement, but it is not responsive to the question.

Passage V (Questions 31–37)

31. According to the passage, commitment is a quality that:

  A. means more to an individual than to a society.
  B. is the root of animal and vegetable life.
  C. is a substructure, not a trait.
  D. has no fundamental underpinnings.

31. C is correct. In paragraph 1 the author says, basically, that commitment is not "just another" trait. Rather, it is a "fundamental underpinning" from which all traits arise. Choice C represents, more or less, the same statement. "Substructure" is intended to *mean the same thing as* "fundamental underpinning."

The wrong answer choices: Choice A is wrong because the passage indicates that commitment is valuable to *both* the individual and the society. Choice B is wrong because the author distinguishes between animal and vegetable life, noting that vegetable life is incapable of commitment. Choice D takes the author's words and distorts their meaning. The author says that commitment *is* a "fundamental underpinning." He does *not* say that commitment lacks fundamental underpinnings.

32. The author states that interpersonal commitment is distinct from societal commitment. From the information in the passage, this statement is probably based on the author's belief that:

   A. interpersonal commitment requires that one person put faith in another.
   B. interpersonal commitment usually leads to intimacy.
   C. societal commitment requires no genuine concern for others.
   D. societal commitment requires no investment.

33. To illustrate a difference between humans and other living things, the author describes the "development of character" (line 11). He wishes to indicate that:

   A. selfhood is attained through commitment to social good.
   B. plants, although living, cannot be said to make commitments.
   C. commitment is essential to the human identity.
   D. human beings are fated to be social beings regardless of their own decisions.

32. **A** is correct. Paragraph 4 presents the relevant text. The author distinguishes interpersonal commitment from societal commitment, noting that one involves devotion to the society and that another involves trust or "investment" in another. Choice A represents, more or less, the same statement.

The wrong answer choices: Choice B takes the author's words and distorts their meaning. The author does not say that interpersonal commitment usually leads to intimacy. He says that it *might* lead to intimacy. Choices C and D are extreme. The word "no" should make you suspicious.

33. **C** is correct. At the beginning of paragraph 2, the author writes that the development of character "depends on commitment." At the end of paragraph 2, he says that commitment "makes us what we are." The paragraph is intended to illustrate that commitment is necessary to a person's identity. That's why C is right.

The wrong answer choices: Choice A sounds "nice." Unfortunately, it does *not* answer the question. Nowhere in paragraph 2 does the author suggest that one's identity depends on commitment to *social good*. Choice B represents a true statement, but it does not represent the author's purpose in comparing humans with other living things. Choice D takes the author's words and distorts their meaning. The author uses the word "social," and he refers to decisions. But he *never* makes any statement like the one set forth in choice D.

34. As described in the passage, Arnold Howe's description of commitment as the sine qua non of social life most probably indicates that:

A. indecision is the cause of most human misery.
B. emotional growth and development are furthered by decision making and commitment.
C. selfhood is attained through devotion to social causes.
D. only humans are capable of programmed genetic development.

34. B is correct. The question requires that you understand the import of paragraph 2. The author and Arnold Howe believe that commitment is the basis on which people develop: It makes them what they are. All you have to do is realize that choice B presents, basically, the same statement. If commitment makes us what we are, it must play an important role in emotional growth and development. It's as simple as that.

The wrong answer choices: Choice A makes an unwarranted statement. The author does not suggest that indecision causes misery. Choice C is also unwarranted. The author says that selfhood is attained through commitment of *various kinds*. Choice D takes the author's words and distorts their meaning. The author refers to genetic programming, but he associates it with *non*human life.

35. Based on the passage, which of the following would most WEAKEN the claim that only humans must make commitments in order to develop their characters?

A. Proof that dogs can reason abstractly.
B. Evidence that animals experience lasting gratification and pain over the need to make choices.
C. Indications that all animals have certain inborn instincts.
D. Documentation that the frontal lobes of some animals are more intricately convoluted than human frontal lobes.

35. B is correct. In paragraph 2, the author associates the importance of commitment with the fact that it may "produce pleasure as it may produce anguish." He says that such pleasure and anguish are the "fabric of character." If it turns out that dogs also experience pain and pleasure over the need to make decisions, then it would begin to appear that commitment plays an important role in *their* development too. It would weaken the author's claim that commitment is important *only* to human development. That's why B is right.

36. It is said that commitment requires persistence. What assertion does the passage make in support of such an idea?

    A. All hobbies require skill that takes years to develop.
    B. People are required to make choices in life.
    C. Seralius continued to write even though he was tortured.
    D. There can be no commitment of energy without a commitment of time.

36. C is correct. If you realize that "persistence" is, more or less, another way of saying "perseverance," you'll turn your attention to paragraph 3. The author discusses the importance of perseverance to social commitment and, as illustration, describes Seralius.

The wrong answer choices: Choices A and D take the author's words and distort their meaning. In paragraph 3 the author refers briefly to hobbies, but he never makes a statement that resembles choice A. Also in paragraph 3, the author refers to "time and energy." But he never says that a commitment of one requires a commitment of the other. He might believe that, but he doesn't say it or suggest it. Choice B accurately reflects the author's view, but it is totally unresponsive to the question.

37. The ability to empathize, according to the passage, is most closely identified with:

    A. increasing openness.
    B. societal commitment.
    C. meaningful intimacy.
    D. the possession of hope.

37. B is correct. In order to answer this question, you have to associate the word "empathize" with the "ability to feel for others," as mentioned in paragraph 3. Once you make that association, it's easy to associate empathy with societal commitment.

The wrong answer choices: Choices A and C take the author's words and distort their meaning. The author discusses intimacy and openness in connection with interpersonal commitment, not societal commitment. Choice D sounds "nice," but the author never refers to hope.

38. The example concerning the small child (lines 25–29) is designed to demonstrate that:

    A. education is more important than freedom.
    B. where people have a meaningful choice between candidates, democracy will succeed.
    C. uninformed voters are easily misled.
    D. education is more easily made equal in a disciplined society.

38. C is correct. After stating that a small child will make decisions that do not conform to her own best interest, the author writes *"Similarly,"* misinformed voters are likely to be duped. In other words, he's saying that misinformed voters are likely to be misled. The discussion of the child is designed to support that point.

The wrong answer choices: Choices A and D take the author's thoughts and distort them. The author believes that education *is important to* freedom. He does not state or imply that it's *more important than* freedom. The author refers to discipline as something a child does not wish to experience. He nowhere posits a relationship between discipline and education, and no such relationship underlies his discussion of the child. Choice B is wrong for the same reason that Choice C is right: The author does not believe that choice *alone* ensures democracy's success.

39. Based on the passage, the government that has the best chance of surviving is:

    A. an oligarchy ruled by a minority.
    B. a democracy whose citizens are well educated.
    C. a well-intentioned monarchy.
    D. a dictatorship.

39. B is correct. The question requires that you put two simple thoughts together. In paragraph 5, the author states that democracy is the strongest of governments. Elsewhere, he plainly indicates that education is necessary to sustain democracy. Simple logic tells you that, according to this author, the government best suited to survive is a democracy with a well-educated populace.

40. The author refers to attempts to foster democracies in underdeveloped nations in order, primarily, to make the point that:

A. no one can govern effectively without understanding the needs of the people.
B. democracy cannot succeed without a well-informed population.
C. education is the most important of all human values.
D. in all forms of government there are those who would seek to gain power by deception.

41. Based on the passage, the view that a democracy vests power "in the people" (lines 16–17) is:

A. widely disbelieved.
B. thoroughly unsupported by historical evidence.
C. a deception that the wealthy perpetrate on the poor.
D. probably unjustified.

40. **B** is correct. In paragraph 3, the author makes the point that democracy requires an educated populace. He notes that democracy fails in underdeveloped nations because the population is *inadequately educated*. His reference to such failed democracies is designed to support the paragraph's central point: Democracy demands education.

The wrong answer choices: Choices A and C are very "nice," but they are wrong. The author does not make or imply the statement represented by choice A or C. The author does not make the statement suggested in choice D, nor is the statement related to the reason for which the author refers to failed attempts at democracy.

41. **D** is correct. The cited lines indicate that democracy does not truly vest power in the people and that it represents a form of oligarchy. Hence, the view that democracy constitutes government by the people is, according to the author, unjustified.

The wrong answer choices: Choice A is wrong because the author nowhere suggests that people generally disbelieve in democracy as a government of the people. Choice B is extreme. The phrase "thoroughly unsupported" should tip you off. Choice C takes the author's words and distorts their meaning. The author suggests that in a democracy, the wealthy tend to hold power, but he does not say that the wealthy trick the poor into believing that *they* have power.

42. According to the passage, most people who wish to spread democracy probably would NOT agree that:

A. education can flourish in the face of poverty.

B. learning depends on physical well-being.

C. poverty must be addressed before learning can proceed.

D. education is a prerequisite to political freedom.

43. The cynic who remarked that "you mustn't enthrone ignorance" (lines 35–37) probably meant that:

A. in a monarchy ignorance has a way of perpetuating itself.

B. ignorant politicians will harm their nations even if they are well meaning.

C. majority rule can be disadvantageous to a public that is not well educated.

D. in a true democracy all people should be entitled to vote regardless of education.

44. Based on information in the passage, one reason that the American government might ultimately deteriorate is that it:

A. is overly concerned with military strength and inadequately concerned with individual rights.

B. strives to offer too much to too many.

C. has not solved the problem of economic inequality.

D. has not dealt appropriately with violence.

---

42. A is correct. The question requires that you put two simple ideas together. In paragraph 2, you're told that democracy requires education. In paragraph 6, you're told that "Most people truly interested in spreading democracy recognize that food, clothing, and shelter are prerequisites to education." People who want to spread democracy realize they must spread education. They also realize that education can't proceed in the face of poverty. Hence, they would *not* believe that democracy can proceed in the face of poverty. That's why A is right.

43. C is correct. The quoted text appears at the end of paragraph 3. The author cites the remark in order to support his point: Democracy requires education. An uneducated voting public will not know how to vote in its own interest.

The wrong answer choices: Choice A is wild and irrelevant. Choice B pertains, somewhat, to paragraph 6 but not to the question at hand. Choice D *runs counter* to the author's attitude.

44. C is correct. The question requires that you associate the phrase "economic inequality" with deprivation of food, clothing, and shelter. Once you make that association, you can deduce from the last paragraph that, in the author's view, democracy is unlikely to survive in an environment of "economic inequality."

45. It may be sensibly inferred from the passage that early industrial capitalists would have regarded the scarcity of material wealth that surrounded them as:

A. positive, because it maintained the class structure to which they were accustomed.
B. positive, because it provided a ready and lucrative market for their products.
C. negative, because it signified an abundance of unmet economic needs.
D. negative, because it diminished opportunities for industrial expansion.

45. B is correct. At the beginning of the second paragraph, you're told that capitalists are not concerned with class but with *sales*. At the end of the paragraph, you're told that material neediness gave capitalists incentive to produce goods that were in demand. Choice B basically restates both those ideas. That's why it's right.

The wrong answer choices: Choices A and C take the author's words and distort their meaning. The author refers to class, but he says that capitalists are *not* concerned with it. The author also refers to unmet economic needs, but he says that such needs provided capitalists with incentive. Choice D is directly opposed to the author's message. The author implies that the scarcity of material wealth *created* opportunities for industrial expansion.

46. One may assume from information in the passage that capitalists profited from improved technology because they were:

A. shrewd in their ability to create demand for the goods they produced.
B. able to increase the availability of goods that were wanted.
C. self-sufficient and hard-working individuals.
D. aware of the need to ameliorate the plight of the poor.

46. B is correct. Paragraph 4 describes improved industrial technologies, and, in view of paragraph 2, it is only natural and right for the reader to assume that the improvements facilitated greater production and profitability.

The wrong answer choices: Choice A "seems" correct, probably because many of us have heard it said that capitalists are shrewd and that they create demand. The author, however, makes no such statement. Choice C sounds "nice," but the author does not refer to capitalists as self-sufficient or hard working. Choice D is wrong because the author never indicates that capitalists are concerned with ameliorating the plight of the poor. We learn that the poor did experience an increase in their standard of living, but it is not stated or suggested that capitalists pursued their activities *in order* that this should happen. Capitalists, we are told, are concerned with *sales*.

47. A reasonable inference from the passage would be that technological advances are attributable in part to:

A. an increased standard of living.
B. market forces.
C. political revolutions based on economic need.
D. freeing individuals from the necessity of performing repetitive work.

47. **B** is correct. The question requires that you associate the phrase "market forces" with demand and the capitalist's desire to *meet* demand. Once you make that association, you realize that these "market forces" created industrialization and that industrialization brought improved technology. Hence, "market forces" contributed to improved technology.

The wrong answer choices: Choice A is unjustified by the passage. Choice C is wild and irrelevant. Choice D takes the author's words and distorts their meaning. The author notes that technology *produced* repetitive work.

48. Implied in the passage is the assumption that advancing technology contributed to:

A. a decreased standard of living for the worker.
B. a longer work day.
C. increased prevalence of consumer services as opposed to consumer goods.
D. loss of the artisan's ability to create, on his own, a complete product.

48. **D** is correct. Although the question uses the word "implied," the matter is explicitly stated in the last paragraph. You're told, specifically, that because of advancing technology, "No one person could produce a whole product." It's as simple as that.

The wrong answer choices: Choices A, B, and C all represent statements that are neither stated nor implied in the passage.

49. The passage asserts that the industrial revolution achieved:

- **A.** better relations between rich and poor.
- **B.** an improved standard of living.
- **C.** increased worker creativity.
- **D.** greater regard for the value of prosperity.

50. The passage states that the industrial revolution produced specialization and automation. It is reasonable to assume that these trends caused:

- I. some people to realize their dreams.
- II. some very large manufacturing companies to become obsolete.
- III. some laborers to work in a way to which they were not accustomed.

- **A.** I only
- **B.** II only
- **C.** I and II only
- **D.** I and III only

51. The passage asserts that furnaces for extracting iron ore greatly increased in size. It is reasonable to conclude that this probably contributed to:

- **A.** decreased use of wood and steel.
- **B.** increased use and production of iron.
- **C.** an overall decrease in industrial wages.
- **D.** a sharp increase in the employment rate.

49. **B** is correct. In paragraph 3, you're told that industrialization "gave rise to . . . [an] increase in the standard of living." Choice B makes, for the most part, the same statement, substituting the word "improved" for "increase in."

The wrong answer choices: Choice A sounds "nice," but the passage describes economic conditions, not "relations." Choice C is contrary to the passage. In paragraph 5, you're told that industrialization created *monotony* in the workplace. Choice D is wild and irrelevant.

50. **D** is correct. The question appears to concern *reasonable assumptions,* but it really asks you to paraphrase text from the passage. In paragraph 5, you're told that many men and women realized their aspirations for material wealth, and you're also told that the nature of their work was permanently transformed. Options I and III, therefore, apply. Option II is contrary to the sense of the passage. You're told that industrialization *created* large manufacturing plants. It did *not* cause them to become obsolete.

51. **B** is correct. The question calls only for common sense and a simple understanding of paragraph 4. You're told that the need to produce in large quantity gave rise to larger industrial apparatus. It stands to simple reason that the larger apparatus, in turn, fostered increased production. Large iron furnaces, therefore, promoted increased use and production of iron.

The wrong answer choices: Choice A is off the point, choice C is unwarranted, and choice D, though not unreasonable, is too emphatic, referring to a "*sharp* increase." Furthermore, choice D is not so closely tied to the passage as is choice B.

Passage VIII (Questions 52–58)

52. The information in the passage is organized according to the:

    A. communal participation in art forms.
    B. enduring quality and value of African art.
    C. varied forms of African art.
    D. influence of geographical region on art form.

53. On the basis of statements made in the passage, one is justified in concluding that the mbari house is largely built to:

    A. honor the gods.
    B. celebrate the Earth.
    C. preserve history.
    D. endure as a religious monument.

52. C is correct. The question requires only that you survey the topics treated by each paragraph and their relationship to one another. Paragraph 1 is introductory and paragraph 4 is conclusory. *Paragraphs 2, 3, and 4 each concern a distinct form of African art.* That's why C is right.

53. A is correct. At the beginning of paragraph 2, you're told that the mbari house "probably represents a religious offering." As soon as you associate the phrase "religious offering" with "honor the gods," you see that A is right.

The wrong answer choices: Choice B takes the author's words and distorts their meaning. You're told that in the front of a mbari house there's often a *figure* of the *goddess* of the Earth. You are not told that the house as a whole is designed to *celebrate* the Earth. Choice C is wholly unjustified and is somewhat contrary to the text. You're told that the house is allowed to deteriorate and that it is not preserved. Choice D also contradicts the text. You're told that the mbari house does not stand as a *lasting* structure. It is allowed to deteriorate.

54. Based on the passage, it is reasonable to conclude that the masks of the Dan tribe differ from those of the Yoruba *Gelade* in that a Dan mask:

- **A.** might accurately describe the role of the person who wears it.
- **B.** is never designed by the person who wears it.
- **C.** has little relationship to social function.
- **D.** is more bewildering in its form.

54. A is correct. In paragraphs 3 and 4, the Dan and Yoruba masks are described. You're told, for example, that in the Dan tribe a judge wears a judge's mask. In the Yoruba group, on the other hand, the masks are used as performance costumes. Hence, in the Dan tribe the mask actually represents the role of the person who wears it. In the Yoruba tribe, it does not. That's why A is right.

The wrong answer choices: Choice B is extreme and irrelevant. The word "never" should tip you off. Choice C is contrary to the text. You're told that the Dan masks do have social function. Choice D is wild.

55. Based on the passage, which of the following would likely characterize the mbari house?

- I. sparse distribution of religiously oriented sculptures.
- II. representations of deities and associated figures.
- III. wear and disrepair.

- **A.** I only
- **B.** II only
- **C.** III only
- **D.** II and III only

55. D is correct. The mbari house is described in paragraph 2. You're told that the mbari house is "filled with" sculptures of deities and that it is never maintained. Hence, II and III apply. Option I is wrong because of the word "sparse," which is nearly opposite to "full" and hence inapplicable.

56. In referring to African art as an "art of life" (paragraph 5), the author probably means that African works of art:

- **A.** are rigorously classified by African artists.
- **B.** include articles used in the course of daily life.
- **C.** are primarily religious in nature.
- **D.** are not valued by the general African public.

56. B is correct. The cited statement is made at the end of the last paragraph, which tells you that African artwork is "not separate from utilitarian objects." African artworks, you are told, include utensils, furniture, clothing, and other items in daily use. The cited statement summarizes that information.

The wrong answer choices: Choice A contradicts the passage. The last paragraph implies that Africans do not view their art in terms of rigid classifications. Choice C represents a statement that is wholly irrelevant to the question, and choice D is wild.

57. It can be reasonably concluded from the passage that the poro are able to manage community affairs largely because their masks:

    I.   command great respect from the tribespeople.
    II. shield their identities.
    III. have little relationship to their function.

   A. I only
   B. II only
   C. I and II only
   D. I, II, and III

57. C is correct. Dan and poro masks are described in paragraph 3. You're told that "community regard" for the masks aids the poro in performing their functions. You're also told that the masks facilitate official action that might be "unpopular" because they afford "anonymity." You'll see that options I and II apply if you associate "community regard" with the phrase "great respect," and "anonymity" with the phrase "shield their identity." Option III is contrary to the passage text. You're told that the poro masks *do* pertain to function.

58. The fact that some art critics insist that all art must be divorced from utilitarian function would most directly challenge the assumption that:

   A. African sculpture has religious significance.
   B. African eating implements constitute art.
   C. Yoruba masks have social significance.
   D. art is best held in collections or museums.

58. B is correct. Although the question refers to "challenging" an "assumption," it requires only simple common sense and knowledge of the word "utilitarian." If one believes that artwork must be divorced from practical use, then one is challenging the notion that an eating implement can constitute art. It's that simple.

59. The writer of the passage seems to believe that Western values:

  A. contribute to tension and hostility among people.
  B. are competitive with Zen values.
  C. produce only unhappiness.
  D. are the product of anxiety and conflict.

59. **A** is correct. In the middle of paragraph 1, you're told that Western values often produce "anxiety, conflict, and combat." The question requires only that you recognize the two statements as being approximately the same.

The wrong answer choices: Choices B and D take the author's words and distort their meaning. The author tells you that Western values are characterized by competition, but he does *not* say that Western values are *in* competition with Zen values. The author says that Western values produce anxiety and conflict. He does *not* say that anxiety and conflict produce Western values. Choice C is extreme. The word "only" should arouse your suspicion.

60. The general point made by the author's comparison of Zen with Western culture is that:

  A. Westerners should incorporate Zen into all facets of their daily lives.
  B. Zen promotes a more natural and tranquil existence than does Western culture.
  C. the drive to succeed usually produces tension and hostility.
  D. Western values are more easily understood than Zen values.

60. **B** is correct. Throughout the passage, the author supports and elaborates his central point set forth in the first paragraph: Zen promotes "peace, humility, and understanding." Western values, on the other hand, foster competition, acquisition, anxiety, conflict, and combat.

The wrong answer choices: Choice A is extreme. The word "all" should set off an alarm. Choice C accurately reflects the author's view, but not his *central point*. Choice D takes the author's thoughts and distorts them. In the first paragraph, the author does suggest that it is difficult to explain Zen values *to a Westerner*, but he nowhere suggests that Zen values are, of themselves, more difficult to understand than Western values.

61. According to the author, Western culture regards mortality as its enemy. The word "enemy" in this context implies that:

    I. Western culture is constantly preoccupied with battle.

    II. Westerners do not accept death as a natural part of life.

    III. Westerners wish to prolong their youth and their lives.

  A. I only
  B. III only
  C. I and II only
  D. II and III only

62. The fact that Hakuin says only, "Is that so," both times he meets the girl's parents is significant because it shows that he:

    I. rejects what the parents are saying to him.

    II. is not concerned with proving himself right or proving others wrong.

    III. is willing to ask questions but never to make assertions.

  A. I only
  B. II only
  C. III only
  D. I, II, and III

63. The passage indicates that a person who does not compete with others probably will:

  A. be satisfied with what he is and what he has.
  B. embrace Western and Zen philosophies alike.
  C. be suspicious of that which appears to have value.
  D. care for others more than he cares for himself.

61. D is correct. Toward the beginning of paragraph 1, the author states that Westerners value youth over age and that they wish to live forever. In characterizing mortality as the "enemy" of Western culture, the author essentially repeats those same points. In order to answer the question, you need only realize that options II and III restate those same points. Option I does not. Rather, it takes the author's words and distorts their meaning.

62. B is correct. The author's point, generally, is that Zen promotes internal peace and that it does not value conquest or confrontation. The story of Hakuin is designed to illustrate the point. Hakuin *accepts*, without attempting to prove himself right or innocent. Option II, therefore, applies. Option I is wild, and Option III is extreme: The word "never" should alert you.

63. A is correct. In paragraph 3, you're told that "One who does not seek to outshine or outdo others has little cause for disappointment." The question requires only that you recognize choice A as a restatement, for the most part, of the same sentiment. "Outshine" and "outdo" signify competition. One who is not disappointed is probably satisfied with what he is and what he has.

The wrong answer choices: Choices B and C are wild. Choice D is "nice," but it doesn't reflect any statement the author has made.

64. The passage indicates that on hearing Hakuin's last statement to them, the father and mother most likely experienced

    I. embarrassment and remorse.
    II. bewilderment.
    III. resentment.

  A. I only
  B. II only
  C. III only
  D. II and III only

65. The author appears to blame the fact that Zen has achieved some reputation for formalism on:

    I. the way in which Zen is represented in China and Japan.
    II. people who claim to follow Zen but do not truly embrace it.
    III. the overbearing character of western culture.

  A. I only
  B. II only
  C. I and II only
  D. I, II, and III

64. **A** is correct. At the very end of the passage, you read that the parents preferred "not to face Hakuin any longer. . . ." That phrase indicates that the parents are feeling embarrassed and somewhat guilty about what they have done. Option I more or less restates that observation. Options II and III are unwarranted.

65. **C** is correct. In paragraph 4, the author notes that Zen has in some places become associated with formalism. In this regard, you're told that some societies have "latched on to the word 'Zen' without adopting its philosophical framework." You're told, specifically, that in China and Japan, Zen is particularly associated with formalism. Hence, options I and II apply. Option III is unwarranted. The author nowhere states or suggests that *western culture* has caused Zen to achieve a reputation for formalism.

Passage I (Questions 1–8)

1. The balanced equation of Reaction II should be:

   A. $2H_2SO_4 + 4Ag \rightarrow 2Ag_2SO_4 + SO_2 + H_2O$.
   B. $2H_2SO_4 + 2Ag \rightarrow Ag_2SO_4 + SO_2 + 2H_2O$.
   C. $3H_2SO_4 + 2Ag \rightarrow Ag_2SO_4 + 2SO_2 + 3H_2O$.
   D. $H_2SO_4 + Ag \rightarrow \frac{1}{2}Ag_2SO_4 + \frac{1}{2}SO_2 + 2H_2O$.

1. **B** is correct. To balance the reaction, you should probably start with Ag_2SO_4.

   Balance the silver:
   $H_2SO_4 + 2Ag \rightarrow Ag_2SO_4 + SO_2 + H_2O$
   Next balance the sulfur:
   $2H_2SO_4 + 2Ag \rightarrow Ag_2SO_4 + SO_2 + H_2O$
   Finally, balance the hydrogen:
   $2H_2SO_4 + 2Ag \rightarrow Ag_2SO_4 + SO_2 + 2H_2O$
   The wrong answer choices: Choices A and D are wrong. Why? A quick glance shows you that some of the elements are unbalanced. For the equation shown in choices A and D, *hydrogen* is unbalanced. For the one shown in choice C, *oxygen* is unbalanced.

2. Which one of the following is a Lewis base?

   A. HSO_4^-
   B. SO_2
   C. SO_3
   D. H_3O^+

2. **A** is correct. This question has nothing to do with the passage. It requires that you review acid-base chemistry and that you remember this: *a Lewis base is a species that donates an electron pair*. Only HSO_4^- has the necessary lone pair available for donation. (You might also answer by noting that HSO_4^- is the conjugate base of the strong acid H_2SO_4.)

   The wrong answer choices: Choices B and C are wrong because the named species don't have a lone pair of electrons, so they can't make the necessary donation. Choice D shows a hydronium which is an acid, not a base.

3. A solution of which two species will most resist a change in the pH when a strong base is added to it?

   A. $Ag_2SO_4 : SO_2$
   B. $H_2SO_4 : SO_3$
   C. $H_2SO_4 : NaHSO_4$
   D. $AgCl : NaCl$

3. **C** is correct. This question should be answered without reference to the passage. Once you review acid-base chemistry, you'll be able to identify a buffer system. A buffer system consists of an acid-base conjugate pair with each member of the pair differing by one proton. Hence, H_2SO_4 and HSO_4^- constitute a buffer system. (Note that Na^+ is a "spectator ion.")

   The wrong answer choices: Choices A, B, and D are wrong because none of the indicated pairs conforms to the specifications of a buffer system.

4. By definition, a Bronsted-Lowry acid is:

   A. any substance capable of acting as a proton acceptor.
   B. any electron-pair acceptor.
   C. any electron-pair donor.
   D. any substance capable of acting as a source of protons.

4. **D** is correct. Once again, the question is answerable without any reference to the passage. By definition, *a Bronsted-Lowry acid is a proton donor,* and choice D paraphrases that definition. It's as simple as that.

   The wrong answer choices: Choice A is wrong because it defines a Bronsted-Lowry *base*. Choice B defines a *Lewis* acid, and choice C defines a Lewis base.

5. Sodium chloride has a higher bond dissociation energy than HCl or H_2O because:

   A. NaCl is of a higher molecular weight than HCl or H_2O.
   B. NaCl is covalently bonded and does not have as great a dipole movement as HCl or H_2O have.
   C. NaCl is not a proton donor like HCl or H_2O.
   D. the electrostatic attractive forces are greater between the ions of NaCl than forces within HCl or H_2O.

5. **D** is correct. When you review chemical bonding, you'll recall that bond dissociation energy is a measure of "bond strength." Your review will also remind you that NaCl has an ionic, electrostatic bond. Such bonds are "strong" and hence have high dissociation energies.

   The wrong answer choices: Choices A and C make true statements, but they don't explain the reported difference in bond dissociation energies. Choice B makes a false statement because NaCl is not *covalently* bonded.

6. An aqueous solution of H_2SO_4 is titrated with a 0.1 M solution of sodium hydroxide, as shown below. Which of the following is true at point 2?

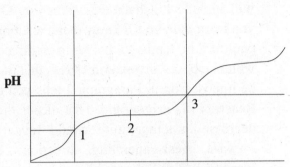

ml of 0.1 M NaOH added

A. The concentration of HSO_4^- equals that of SO_4^{-2}.
B. The major species in solution are Na^+ and HSO_4^-.
C. The pH is equal to the acid dissociation constant of H_2SO_4.
D. Point 2 is the first equivalence point.

7. At a temperature of 350°C and a pressure of 320 atm, a sample of 1 mole of H_2SO_4 has completely dissociated into gaseous SO_3 and H_2O. Approximately what is the ratio of the velocities of these two molecules? (M.W. of SO_3 is 80 g/mol.)

A. $2\sqrt{3}$
B. $\dfrac{3\sqrt{2}}{2}$
C. $1\sqrt{5}$
D. $\dfrac{3\sqrt{5}}{10}$

6. **B** is correct. This question requires that you become familiar with acid-base titration curves. Once you do, you'll see that point 2 on the graph $[HSO_4^-] = [SO_4^{-2}]$.

The wrong answer choices: Choice A is wrong because at point 2, no H_2SO_4 remains. Choice C is wrong because at point 2, the pKa of HSO_4^- (not H_2SO_4), equals the pH. Choice D is wrong because point 2 is not an equivalence point. (Points 1 and 3 are equivalence points.)

7. **B** is correct. The question gives you more information than you need to answer it. After you've learned (or relearned) something about so-called Kinetic-Molecular theory, you'll know that the ratio of the velocities of 2 molecules is inversely proportional to the square root of the ratio of their masses:

$$V_{H_2O} / V_{SO_3} = (M_{SO_3}/M_{H_2O})^{1/2} =$$
$$(80/18)^{1/2} = \text{approx. } (81/18)^{1/2}$$
$$(81/18)^{1/2} = (9/2)^{1/2} = 3/(2)^{1/2} = 3(2)^{1/2} / 2$$

8. Assuming Reaction I is at equilibrium, which of the following changes will cause an increase in the concentration of sulfuric acid?

   A. Decreasing the pressure
   B. Decreasing the concentration of SO_3
   C. The addition of a catalyst
   D. Decreasing the temperature

8. **D** is correct. The question requires that you look closely not only at Reaction I but also at paragraph 2. Your review of chemistry will include LeChatalier's principle. Once you learn *that*, you'll know that a reaction at equilibrium tends to move in a direction which opposes any external stress that might be imposed on it. Paragraph 2 tells you that Reaction I is *exothermic*. That means that a decrease in temperature would favor the forward, heat-generating direction. The formation of H_2SO_4 would increase.

The wrong answer choices: Choice A is wrong because decreased pressure would favor the reverse direction, which will tend to restore pressure. Choice B is wrong for pretty much the same reason: A decrease in the amount of reactant also favors the reverse direction, which will tend to restore the concentration of reactant. Choice C is wrong because a catalyst increases the *rate* at which equilibrium is reached, but it does not change equilibrium *concentrations*.

Passage II (Questions 9–16)

9. A particle is fired into the magnetic field. Its initial velocity has components along path Y and into the page. The angle the particle's velocity vector makes with path Y is called phi. Phi can assume values between 0 and $\frac{\pi}{2}$. Which of the following graphs best represents the dependence of the magnitude of the force on the particle to angle phi?

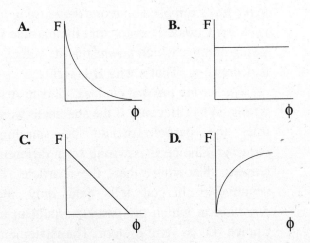

A.

B.

C.

D.

10. Keeping all other factors constant, what changes could be made so particle X traveled in a larger spiral?

   A. Increase the density of the magnetic field.
   B. Give the particle more kinetic energy.
   C. Give the particle less kinetic energy.
   D. Increase the charge on the particle.

9. **A** is correct. The question tests your ability to recognize a graphic expression of a relationship that's been described in words. Careful consideration of the diagram reveals the following relationship: $\theta + \phi = \pi/2$. If you apply this information to the formula set forth in the passage, you realize:

F = Bqv sin ($\pi/2 - \phi$)

F = -Bqv sin ($\phi - \pi/2$)

F = Bqv cos (ϕ)

The graph in choice A shows the same relationship.

The wrong answer choices: Choices B and C are wrong because neither reveals a trigonometric curve. Choice D is wrong because it contradicts the formula described in the passage. It indicates that F would be *smallest* when perpendicular to the magnetic field. F would be *greatest* when parallel to it.

10. **B** is correct. The question can be answered by process of elimination. One could increase the spiral's size either by decreasing the force on the particle (the particle wouldn't turn so *much)*, or increasing the particle's velocity (the particle wouldn't turn so *fast)*. Increasing kinetic energy *means* increasing velocity. That's why B is right.

The wrong answer choices: Choices A and D are wrong since pursuing the measures they describe would increase the force on the particle and make the spiral *tighter*. Choice C is wrong because reducing the particle's kinetic energy would also make the spiral tighter.

11. Particle Z is given an initial velocity of 1×10^3 m/s along path Y. If the field density is 5.5 T and particle Z has a charge of 1 coul, how strong will the net force on the particle be when it first enters the field?

A. 0 N
B. 5.5×10^3 N
C. 1.1×10^3 N
D. 2.5×10^3 N

11. **B** is correct. Take the values provided in the question and plug them into the equation described in the passage:

$$F = Bqv \sin\theta$$
$$F = (5.5 \text{ T})(1 \text{ coul})(1 \times 10^3 \text{ m/sec})$$
$$(\sin 90°)$$
$$F = 5.5 \times 10^3 \text{ N}$$

12. Particle X spirals inward instead of revolving around a fixed point because:

A. the particle's velocity is increasing.
B. the particle is losing energy.
C. the particle is negatively charged.
D. the net force on the particle is perpendicular to the plane formed by its velocity vector and the direction of the magnetic field.

12. **B** is correct. The fact that the particle is spiraling inward implies either an *increase in the force* imposed on it or a *decrease in its velocity*. Choice B states that the particle is losing energy, which *means* that its velocity is decreasing. That's why B is right.

The wrong answer choices: Choice A is wrong. Why? Because if the statement were true, the particle would be spiraling *outward*. Choice C is wrong for a different reason. Knowing that the particle is negatively charged tells you only the *direction* in which the particle would turn. Choice D is wrong, too. The statement explains why the particle travels in circular motion, but it doesn't explain, specifically, why it spirals *inward*.

13. If particle P were also given a velocity component into the page equal to the magnitude of its velocity in the direction of path Y, the force first felt by the particle would:

A. decrease by a factor of $\dfrac{2}{\sqrt{2}}$.

B. decrease by a factor of $\dfrac{1}{\sqrt{2}}$.

C. remain the same.

D. increase by a factor of $\sqrt{2}$.

13. **C** is correct. First you have to pay attention to the fact that P's velocity component is *into the page*, which means that it's parallel to the direction of the magnetic field. Then you use the equation given to you in the passage; angle θ, which is between the direction of the particle's velocity and the magnetic field, would be zero. That means the force is zero. Hence, an additional velocity component into the page adds no additional component of force.

14. Assume the magnetic field density is 5.5 T. A large charged object of mass 1 kg and charge 1 coul is sent into the magnetic field along path Y. How fast would the object have to be traveling so the force of the magnetic field and the force of gravity were in equilibrium?

    A.   0.6 m/s
    B.   1.8 m/s
    C.   5.4 m/s
    D.   2.7 m/s

15. A particle of mass .001 kg and charge 1 coul enters the magnetic field traveling 1000 m/s. The particle spirals and comes to a complete stop relative to the field in 0.05 s. How much work was done by the magnetic field? Neglecting the force of gravity, this event represents work equal to:

    A.   20 J
    B.   25 J
    C.   500 J
    D.   10000 J

16. The following diagrams represent the path of a negative test charge moving from point A to point B inside the electric field produced by a negatively charged particle. Which path requires the most amount of work to move the test charge?

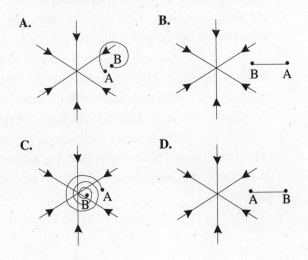

14. **B** is correct. Since the magnetic and gravitational forces are in equilibrium, they must be equal:

$$Bqv \sin\theta = mg$$
$$(5.5\ \text{T})(1\ \text{coul})\ v\ (\sin 90°) =$$
$$(1\ \text{kg})(9.8\ \text{m/sec}^2)$$
$$v = 1.8\ \text{m/sec}$$

15. **C** is correct. Once you review the concepts of work and energy, you'll know that work is equivalent to change in kinetic energy, and you'll realize that:

$$W = \Delta KE = KE_{initial} - KE_{final}$$
$$W = (1/2)mv^2 - 0\ \text{J}$$
$$W = (1/2)(.001\ \text{kg})(1000\ \text{m/sec})^2$$
$$W = 500\ \text{J}$$

16. **B** is correct. This question has nothing to do with the passage. It requires that you review the subject of work and energy and take special note of the fact that work is independent of path. That means that when you're talking about work, displacement is relevant, but distance isn't. Since both charges are negative, they can't come together unless work is done on them. Naturally, more work is necessary to close a gap of relatively greater size than to close a gap of relatively smaller size. Among the choices, B represents closure of the largest gap. That's why it's right.

The wrong answer choices: Choices A and C are wrong. Although the figures describe long paths between A and B, they also show that A and B ultimately find themselves close together. Choice D is wrong because it would indicate that a *negative* quantity of work is performed. (Actually, Choice A is also wrong for that reason.)

17. Which of the following events in a synthesis reaction describes a decrease in entropy?

    A. The number of moles of product is more than the number of moles of reactants.
    B. The number of moles of product is less than the number of moles of reactants.
    C. The phase of the reactants is more ordered than the phase of the product.
    D. The phase of the reactants is more structured than the phase of the product.

18. The heat lost or gained during the breakage and reformation of bonds between atoms in a synthesis reaction is:

    A. Gibbs' free energy.
    B. Helmholtz free energy.
    C. kinetic energy.
    D. heat of reaction.

17. **B** is correct. You can answer the question without regard to the passage. Your review of thermodynamics will remind you that entropy is a measure of "disorder." If for some reaction there are fewer moles of product on the right than there are moles of reactant on the left side, the reaction represents an increase in order and entropy *decreases*.

The wrong answer choices: Choices A, C, and D all describe situations in which the left side of the equation shows relatively greater order. That means the forward reaction would lead to greater disorder, and hence to an *increase* in entropy.

18. **D** is correct. After you learn or relearn thermodynamics, you'll realize that the "heat lost or gained during the breakage and reformation of bonds between atoms in a synthesis reaction" *means* "heat of reaction" (which is also known as enthalpy change). Remember, also, that if a reaction produces a net heat gain, it's *endothermic*. If it produces a net heat loss, it's *exothermic*.

The wrong answer choices: Choice A is wrong because Gibbs' free energy is a function of enthalpy *and* entropy. Choice B is wrong because Helmholtz free energy (which you *don't* have to understand for the MCAT) is also a function of entropy. Choice C is wrong because *kinetic* energy is energy of *motion*.

19. According to Table 2, the formation of $CO_2(g)$ from elemental carbon and oxygen proceeds spontaneously because:

A. the reaction produces a net gain in stability.
B. the reaction produces a net loss in stability.
C. the reaction produces a net gain in entropy.
D. the reaction produces a net gain in enthalpy.

19. **A** is correct. The reaction will occur spontaneously only if it tends to increase stability.

The wrong answer choices: Choice B is wrong because decreased stability means that a reaction is *not* spontaneous. Choices C and D can be eliminated quickly. Think about the reaction they describe:

$$C(s) + O_2(g) \rightarrow CO_2(g)$$

Entropy is *decreasing,* and there's a loss of enthalpy.

20. What is the approximate mass of $FeCl_2$ contained in a 1.0 liter of 0.7 molar solution of $FeCl_2$?

A. 64 g
B. 88 g
C. 130 g
D. 180 g

20. **B** is correct. This is a straightforward stoichiometry problem. The molecular weight of $FeCl_2$ is $55.8 + 71 = 126.8$ g/mol. In 1.0 liter of a 0.7 molar solution of $FeCl_2$, there are 0.7 mole of $FeCl_2$. The 0.7 mole of $FeCl_2$ is equivalent to 0.7 mole $\times$ (126.8 g/mole), or 88 grams of $FeCl_2$.

21. If a particular synthesis proceeds spontaneously, which of the following should be anticipated?

A. ΔG is positive; ΔH is negative.
B. ΔG is positive; ΔH is positive.
C. ΔG is negative; ΔH is negative.
D. ΔG is negative; ΔH is positive.

21. **C** is correct. If a reaction is spontaneous, Gibbs' free energy is negative. Once you review kinetics, you'll know that:

$$\Delta G = \Delta H - T\Delta S$$

H is the enthalpy; T is the temperature; and S is the entropy. For a spontaneous reaction, ΔH is negative since it makes a negative contribution to the value of ΔG.

The wrong answer choices: Choices A and B are wrong because a positive ΔG means that the reaction is not spontaneous. Choice D is not as good as C because a positive ΔH would tend to make ΔG more positive and less spontaneous.

22. When 1 mole of $Fe_2O_3(c)$ and 1 mole of $N_2O_4(g)$ are formed from their constituent elements, how much energy is supplied or released to the environment?

    A. 815.0 kJ/mol gained
    B. 815.0 kJ/mol lost
    C. 833.4 kJ/mol gained
    D. 833.4 kJ/mol lost

23. The investigator determined the specific heat of the two compounds, Fe and H_2O. For Fe the value was 0.5 J/g°C, and for H_2O the value was 4.0 J/g°C. If the investigator added 8 g of Fe at 60°C to 99 g of water at 30°C, what would be the temperature of the resulting mixture?

    A. -29.7°C
    B. 0.0°C
    C. 30.3°C
    D. 40.1°C

22. **B** is correct. Table 1 provides the relevant enthalpy values. When 1 mole of Fe_2O_3 is formed, 824.2 kJ of heat are lost, and when 1 mole of N_2O_4 is formed, 9.2 kJ are gained. Considered together, the two reactions produce:

824.2 kJ lost − 9.2 kJ gained = 815 kJ lost.

23. **C** is correct. After reviewing thermochemistry, you'll know how to solve this kind of problem. For this situation, the amount of heat gained equals the amount of heat lost. The amount of heat gained or lost, Q, is equal to the (mass of the species) × (specific heat) × (change in temperature).

1. $Q_{lost} = Q_{gained}$
2. $m_{Fe}(0.5 J/g°C)(60°C - T_{final}) =$
    $M_{H_2O}(4.0 J/g°C)(T_{final} - 30°C)$
3. $(8 g)(0.5 J/g°C)(60°C - T_{final}) =$
    $(99g)(4.0 J/g°C)(T_{final} - 30°C)$
4. $240 - 4T_{final} = 396T_{final} - 11880$
5. $12120 = 400T_{final}$
6. $T_{final} = 1212/40 = 30.3°C$

The wrong answer choices: Choices A and B should be eliminated quickly. If one mixes two substances, he cannot produce a mixture with a temperature that is lower than that of either one. Choice D is a trap. You'd arrive at the answer if you'd forgotten to designate the change in temperature of the iron as $60°C - T_{final}$.

Passage IV (Questions 24–29)

24. Two particles travel through a magnetic field. If the first particle experiences a net force and the second particle is unaffected, which of the following particles are they?

   A. Beta and alpha
   B. Gamma and neutrino
   C. Beta and neutrino
   D. Gamma and alpha

24. **C** is correct. After reviewing electricity and magnetism, you'll remember that charged particles traveling through a magnetic field experience a force. After you review radioactive decay, you'll know which decay products are charged and which are not. Since beta particles carry a negative charge, they experience a force when moved through a magnetic field. Since neutrinos are uncharged, they don't.

   The wrong answer choices: Choices B and D are wrong because each lists as its first particle a gamma ray. Gamma rays are *un*charged. A is wrong because it lists as its second particle an alpha particle. Alpha particles have a net *positive* charge.

25. Two helium nuclei fuse and release energy in the form of photons. Which of the following describes the main energy transfer that takes place?

   A. Kinetic to kinetic
   B. Electrical to kinetic
   C. Mass to electromagnetic
   D. Kinetic to electrical

25. **C** is correct. This question has nothing to do with the passage. It requires that you review nuclear reactions and remember that fusion reactions convert mass to energy.

   The wrong answer choices: A, B, and D should be eliminated because photons are electromagnetic waves.

26. $^{236}_{90}$Th emits two beta particles and two alpha particles. Which of the following nuclei results?

   A. $^{226}_{87}$Fr   B. $^{226}_{88}$Ra

   C. $^{228}_{88}$Ra   D. $^{224}_{86}$Rn

26. **C** is correct. To answer this question you write this equation:

$$^{236}_{90} \xrightarrow{\enspace \textcircled{2\beta} \enspace} {}^{236}_{92} \xrightarrow{\enspace \textcircled{2\alpha} \enspace} {}^{m}_{n}$$

The atomic *numbers* must be in balance:

$$90 = n + (2)(-1) + (2)(2)$$
$$n = 88$$

Look on the periodic table for element 88:

$$X = Ra.$$

The atomic *weights* also must be in balance:

$$236 = m + (2)(0) + (2)(4)$$
$$m = 228$$

The answer must be Ra-228.

27. Half of a sample of Tl will decay to Pb in 3.1 mins through the emission of beta particles. If an initially pure sample of Tl contains 7 g of lead after 9.3 mins, what was the approximate mass of the original sample?

   A.   7 g
   B.   8 g
   C.   28 g
   D.   32 g

27. **B** is correct. Once you review radioactive decay, you'll realize that this is a simple MCAT half-life problem. You should ignore the reference to beta decay and answer the question without regard to the passage.

9.3 mins is the same as 3 half-lives.

After three half-lives, 7/8 of the substance will have decayed:

$$(7/8)x = 7 \text{ g}$$
$$x = 8 \text{ g}$$

The wrong answer choices: Choice A should be eliminated right away. If the statement were true, all of the substance would have decayed. In an MCAT half-life problem, that can't happen. Choices C and D are wrong.

28. An element decays to an isotope of itself, releasing alpha and beta particles. The number of alpha particles to beta particles would have to be in the ratio of:

A. $\frac{1}{2}$

B. 1

C. 2

D. 4

28. A is correct. Because the element decayed to an isotope *of itself*, its atomic *number* is constant. Alpha decay *decreases* the atomic number by two. Beta decay increases atomic number by one. Atomic number will be constant only if there are two beta decays for every alpha decay.

29. If 2.8 MeV are needed to produce 1 photon, how many photons can be produced when 1 gram of matter is converted to energy?

A. 2×10^{26}
B. 2×10^{32}
C. 2×10^{35}
D. 4×10^{35}

29. A is correct. Photons have energy but no mass. When you read about converting mass to energy you should remember Einstein's formula:

$$E = mc^2$$
$$E = (.001 \text{ kg})(3 \times 10^8 \text{ m/s})^2$$
$$E = 9 \times 10^{13} \text{ J}$$

Now you have to figure out how many photons correspond to this particular quantity of energy:

$$(9 \times 10^{-13} \text{ J})(1 \text{ photon/ } 2.8 \text{ MeV}) \times$$
$$(1 \text{ eV}/1.6 \times 10^{-19} \text{ J})(1 \text{ MeV}/10^6 \text{ eV}) =$$
$$2 \times 10^{26} \text{ photons}$$

The wrong answer choices: Choice B is a trap. You arrive at that number if you forget to convert grams to kilograms. Choice C is another trap. You'd reach that number if you forgot to convert MeV to eV. Choice D is not a trap. It's just wrong, plain and simple.

30. Light traveling through water in a swimming pool has the following measured values:

frequency = 5×10^{14} Hz

phase angle = $\dfrac{\pi}{2}$

wavelength = 4.5×10^{-7} m
velocity = 2.25×10^{8} m/s

The wave propagates across the surface of the water into air. If the speed of light in air is 3×10^{8} m/s, what is the frequency of the wave traveling in air?

A. 2.5×10^{14} Hz
B. 3.8×10^{14} Hz
C. 5.0×10^{14} Hz
D. 6.7×10^{14} Hz

31. A trigonal bipyramid is the characteristic of the orbital geometry of an atom in which hybridization?

A. sp
B. sp^2
C. sp^3
D. dsp^3

32. Which of the following electronic configurations belongs to a diamagnetic element in its ground state?

A. $1s^2 2s^1$
B. $1s^2 2s^2 2p^1$
C. $1s^2 2s^2 2p^4$
D. $1s^2 2s^2 2p^6$

30. **C** is correct. Once you review waves, you'll recall that wave velocity is the product of frequency and wavelength. You'll also know that when a light wave passes from one medium to another its wavelength or velocity might change, but its frequency does not. So the whole matter is really quite simple. The wave equation applies and the wave's frequency in the air is equal to its frequency in the water.

31. **D** is correct. After you review hybridized bonding you'll know that a trigonal bipyramid structure requires the availability of *five* hybrid orbitals. Among the configurations listed in the choices, only dsp^3 fulfills this requirement. The number of pure orbitals contributing to hybridization equals the total number of hybrid orbitals finally formed.

The wrong answer choices: Choices A, B, and C provide only 2-, 3-, and 4-hybrid orbitals, respectively.

32. **D** is correct. Diamagnetic elements have no unpaired electrons, and that's the situation reflected in choice D.

The wrong answer choices: Choices A and B are wrong because they show an *odd* number of electrons, which means that some electrons must be unpaired. Choice C is wrong even though it shows an even number of electrons. When you review orbital filling and electron configuration, you'll revisit Hund's rule: There must be two unpaired electrons in the p orbital.

33. Three mechanical waves of frequencies 3 Hz, 5 Hz, and 7 Hz are passed through the same medium at equal velocities. The magnitudes of their respective displacement are 1, 2, and 4. What is the smallest possible displacement in the medium that could be caused by the resultant wave?

    A.   0
    B.   1
    C.   7
    D.   8

33. **B** is correct. The superposition of any number of waves with differing frequencies and amplitudes will result in a *complex* wave. To solve this problem, you need to add the displacements caused by individual waves at each point in such a way as to create the smallest possible resulting displacement. (Or it could be the greatest possible destruction.) This will result from adding: $4 - (1 + 2) = 1$.

34. Which of the following is true when comparing Be and Cl?

    A.   The electronegativity of Cl is much less than that of Be.
    B.   The electron affinity of Cl is much less than that of Be.
    C.   The atomic radius of the atom Cl is much larger than that of the atom Be.
    D.   Cl is not very reactive, whereas Be, an alkaline Earth metal, is reactive.

34. **C** is correct. A review of periodic trends will tell you that (1) electronegativity and electron affinity are greatest for elements in the upper-right-hand portion of the periodic table and (2) atomic radius is greatest for elements in the lower-left part of the table. Since chlorine's valence electrons are located in the third energy level, its radius is larger than that of berillium.

   The wrong answer choices: Choice A, B, and D are wrong, and once again, a review of periodic trends tells you why. Chlorine requires only one electron to complete its outermost shell. Therefore it has high electronegativity, electron affinity, and chemical reactivity.

35. What pH would most likely cause a color change in the unknown indicator?

   A. 5
   B. 7
   C. 9
   D. 14

35. **A** is correct. In the last two sentences of the passage, you're told that the color change occurred at a pH below the equivalence pH of 7.0. Among the choices, only A represents a pH below 7.0.

36. Which of the following colors would result from the formation of the conjugate base of bromothymol blue?

   A. Spectral red
   B. Blue
   C. Yellow
   D. Green

36. **B** is correct. In paragraph 1 of the passage you learn that the conjugate base (In_B^-) of bromothymol blue is—blue.
   The wrong answer choices: Choices A and D refer to colors not mentioned in paragraph 1 or in connection with bromothymol blue. Choice C is wrong because yellow is the color of the *acid* form of the indicator (HIn_A).

37. At pH 7.0, the solution's color most probably indicates the presence of:

   A. HIn_A^-

   B. In_A^-

   C. In_B^-

   D. HIn_B^-

37. **C** is correct. The indicator is in its conjugate base form at pH just below pH 7.0. Hence, it has the symbol In_B^-.
   The wrong answer choices: Choice A is wrong because the indicated symbol denotes the *acid* form of the indicator. Choices B and D are wrong because the indicated symbols are not used or defined in the passage. They don't really mean anything.

38. Two additional indicators were used. For HCl, phenolphthalein changed color above the equivalence point, and methyl red changed color below the equivalence point. At the equivalence point, which forms of the indicators produce color?

   A. The base of phenolphthalein and the acid of methyl red
   B. The base of methyl red and the acid of phenolphthalein
   C. The acids of both indicators
   D. The bases of both indicators

38. **B** is correct. Methyl red changes color below the equivalence point. *At* the equivalence point, it is present in conjugate base form. Phenolphthalein changes color above the equivalence point, and *at* the equivalence point, remains in its acid form.

39. The color change of the unknown indicator represented a shift of the equilibrium reaction $HIn_A \longleftrightarrow H^+ + In_B^-$:

A. to the ground state configuration.
B. to formation of the conjugate acid.
C. to the left.
D. to the right.

40. According to the information below, which of the following indicators will be present in the acid form in an aqueous titration solution that reached pH 5.0?

Indicator	Acid	Base Color	K_{ind} Color	pH Range
Thymol blue	Red	Yellow	2×10^{-2}	1.2 – 2.8
Methyl orange	Red	Orange	3.5×10^{-4}	3.1 – 4.4
Bromothymol blue	Yellow	Blue	8×10^{-8}	6.0 – 7.6

A. Thymol blue, because the conjugate acid remains protonated at the pH value of the solution
B. Thymol blue, because the conjugate base is deprotonated at the pH value of the solution
C. Bromothymol blue, because the conjugate acid remains protonated at the pH value of the solution
D. Bromothymol blue, because the conjugate base is deprotonated at the pH value of the solution

39. **D** is correct. The necessary information is in the last paragraph. As OH^- is added, protons are removed, and the reaction shifts to the right.

The wrong answer choices: Choice A is wild and irrelevant. Choices B and C are really saying the same thing. A shift to the left represents formation of the conjugate acid. Choices B and C can't *both* be right, so both should be eliminated.

40. **C** is correct. The right-hand column of the table describes the pH range at which each indicator is converted to its conjugate base form. At pH 5, bromothymol blue is not yet converted. It remains in its *acid* form.

The wrong answer choices: Choices A and B should be eliminated. The table shows you that well below pH 5, thymol blue is completely converted to its conjugate base form. Choice D is wrong because it contradicts the question.

41. The piston is pulled upward so that the new fluid heights in stems A and B are h_1 and h_2, respectively. Which of the following relate h_0, h_1, and h_2?

    A. $h_0 < h_1 < h_2$
    B. $h_1 < h_0 < h_2$
    C. $h_2 < h_0 < h_1$
    D. $h_0 = h_2 < h_1$

41. **C** is correct. Consider the figure. There's a vacuum in Stem A, in between the liquid surface and the piston. When the piston rises, the fluid in stem A rises too—to h_1. The fluid height in stem B must drop to h_2. Assuming that fluid remains in stem B and does not drop below h_0, h_1 *must* be greatest, and h_0 lowest.

42. If both stems A and B have fluid at height h_0, what is the difference in pressure between points x and y? (Assume atmospheric pressure is 1.013×10^5 Pa.)

    A. 5.0×10^3 Pa
    B. 1.0×10^5 Pa
    C. 1.5×10^5 Pa
    D. 2.5×10^5 Pa

42. **A** is correct. The difference in pressure, ΔP, between two points in stagnant fluid is $\rho g \Delta h$. ρ is the density of the fluid, g is the acceleration due to gravity, and Δh is the difference in height between the two points. So:

$$\Delta P = (5.0 \times 10^3 \text{kg/m}^3)(10\text{m/s}^2)(0.1\text{m})$$
$$= 5 \times 10^3 \text{ Pa}$$

43. If the piston is moved such that the height of the fluid in stem A is lowered by 20% of its initial height, h_0, what is the work done on the fluid in terms of h_0 and π? (Use 10 m/s^2 for the value of gravitational acceleration.)

    A. $\pi (h_0)/10$ J
    B. $5\pi (h_0)^2$ J
    C. $2\pi \times 10^7 h_0$ J
    D. $25\pi \times 10^5/h_0$ J

43. **B** is correct. If the height of fluid in stem A is lowered by 20 percent (0.2) of its initial height, h_0, the piston must move downward as well. The height of the fluid in stem B increases by 0.2 of *its* initial height, h_0. To ascertain the associated *work,* we use the formula provided in the passage:

W = $\Delta P \Delta V$

$$\Delta P = pg \, \Delta h$$
$$= (5 \times 10^3 \text{ kg/m}^3)(10 \text{ m/s}^2)(0.2 h_0 \text{ m})$$
$$= h_0 \times 10^4 \text{kg/ms}^2$$
$$\Delta V = \pi r^2 \Delta h$$
$$= \pi (0.05 \text{ m})^2 (0.2 h_0 \text{ m})$$
$$= 5\pi h_0 \times 10^{-4} \text{ m}^3$$

$$W = \Delta P \, \Delta V = 5\pi h_0^2 \, \frac{Rgm^2}{s^2} = 5\pi h_0^2 \text{ J}$$

44. The piston is removed and the liquid reaches a height of 20 m in each stem. A small hole appears at point y, and a steady flow of fluid escapes. Ignoring friction, what is the velocity at which fluid leaves the U-tube? (Use 10 m/s^2 for the value of gravitational acceleration.)

    A. 10 m/s
    B. 12 m/s
    C. 17 m/s
    D. 20 m/s

44. **D** is correct. Once you review Bernoulli's equation and Toricelli's theorem, you'll know that a fluid's velocity equals:

the square root of
(2g × the height of the fluid above)
Velocity=$(2 \times 10 \text{ m/s}^2 \times 20 \text{ m})^{1/2}$=20 m/s

Passage VII (Questions 45–50)

45. The dependence of the viscosity and surface tension of water on temperature is best illustrated by which of the following figures?

A.
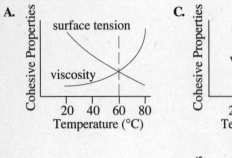

C.
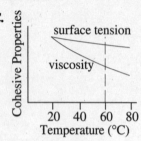

B.
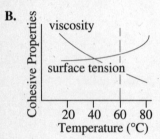

D.
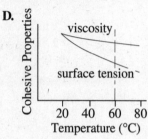

46. Which phenomenon accounts for the decrease in density of water as its temperature decreases from 4°C to 0°C?

A. Hydrogen bonding in the liquid phase
B. Covalent bonds formed in the gas phase
C. Covalent bonds in the closed lattice
D. Hydrogen bonding in the open lattice

45. **C** is correct. The important information is in paragraph 3. You're told that from 20°C to 60°C, viscosity decreases by more than 50 percent, while surface tension decreases by only 5 percent. Choice C shows a graph wherein viscosity decreases much more quickly than does surface tension.

The wrong answer choices: A and B should be eliminated because each of the graphs they present shows a cohesive property becoming more pronounced with *increase* in temperature. That doesn't happen. Choice D is wrong because it shows surface tension falling more quickly than viscosity in the range of 20°C to 60°C.

46. **D** is correct. Paragraph 2 of the passage tells you that hydrogen bonding produces the open lattice structure of solid water.

The wrong answer choices: Choices A and B should be eliminated because at 0°C and 4°C water is in the solid phase only (assuming normal pressure). Choice C is wrong because the passage and question concern *open* lattice structure. Closed lattice is not mentioned.

47. When ice melts at 0°C, what enthalpy change occurs during the formation of the liquid phase under standard equilibrium conditions?

A. The reaction releases 6.008 kJ/mol.
B. The reaction consumes 6.008 kJ/mol.
C. The reaction releases 44.02 kJ/mol.
D. The reaction equilibrium results in 44.94 kJ/mol energy release.

47. **B** is correct. The question requires that you (1) read the table effectively and (2) know that when water melts, heat must be absorbed or consumed.

The wrong answer choices: Choices A, C, and D should be eliminated because heat cannot possibly be *released* as ice melts.

48. A water molecule is able to form hydrogen bonds because of its:

A. ability to form a crystalline lattice at vaporization.
B. ability to form ionic bonds, as measured by ionization energy.
C. ability to form covalent bonds, as measured by its electron affinity.
D. degree of polarity, as measured by the dipole moment.

48. **D** is correct. The question is unrelated to the passage. Your review of bonding will remind you that only oxygen, nitrogen, and fluorine form hydrogen bonds because they form molecules with large dipole moments.

The wrong answer choices: Choices A and B are wrong because they make false statements. There are no crystalline structures at vaporization temperatures, and water does not form ionic bonds. Choice C is wrong because covalent bonding does not explain how or why water forms hydrogen bonds.

49. The volume of 1.00 g of water at 4°C under standard pressures is less than the volume of 1.00 g of water at 25°C.

These results confirm that water at 25°C:

A. has a lower density.
B. has a higher vapor pressure.
C. has a greater molecular weight.
D. undergoes ionization.

49. **A** is correct. The question requires that you know the meaning of density in mathematical terms. Density is mass per volume. If mass is constant, decreased volume means increased density; increased volume means decreased density.

The wrong answer choices: Choice B represents a true statement, but it doesn't explain how 1.00 g of water experiences a change in volume with a change in temperature. Choice C is wrong because water has only *one* molecular formula and one molecular weight. Such things *don't change*. Choice D is wrong because ionization has no bearing on change in volume.

50. The hybrid orbitals in a water molecule are correctly identified by which of the following?

   A. 4 sp^3 orbitals in a trigonal array with two nonbonding pairs of electrons
   B. 4 sp^3 orbitals in a tetrahedral array with two nonbonding pairs of electrons
   C. 4 sp^2 orbitals in a trigonal array with two nonbonding pairs of electrons
   D. 3 sp^2 orbitals in a tetrahedral array with three nonbonding pairs of electrons

50. **B** is correct. After you review Lewis structures and hybridization, you'll be able to sketch the Lewis structure of water. Oxygen has six valence electrons, and each hydrogen atom has one valence electron. Hence, the Lewis structure must account for a total of eight valence electrons. The sketch should look like:

$$H:\ddot{\underset{..}{O}}:H$$

After you review hybridized bonding, you'll see that the oxygen atom has two lone pairs of electrons and two sigma bonds. The oxygen has a structure number of 4 and undergoes sp^3 hybridization. The four hybrid orbitals produce a tetrahedron.

51. Within the orbital structure of an atom, as the second quantum number (l) increases, the number of orbitals:

   A. increases according to $2l$.
   B. increases according to $2l + 1$.
   C. increases according to l.
   D. remains the same.

51. B is correct. When you study quantum numbers, you'll learn that an electron's first quantum number represents a shell and that its second quantum number represents a *sub*shell. For any subshell, there are $2l + 1$ orbital shapes, all having equal energy. $l = 0$ represents the s subshell, and there's one s subshell per shell. $l = 1$ represents the p orbital, and there are $3p$ orbitals per shell (beginning with the second shell). $l = 2$ represents the d orbital, and there are three $5d$ = orbitals per shell (-2, -1, 0, 1, 2), beginning with the third shell.

52. A car of mass m is rolling down a ramp that is elevated at an angle of 60°. What is the magnitude of the car's acceleration parallel to the ramp?

   A. $\dfrac{mg\sqrt{3}}{3}$

   B. $\dfrac{\sqrt{3}g}{2}$

   C. $\dfrac{g}{2}$

   D. $\dfrac{2g}{3}$

52. B is correct. A review of basic trigonometry will give you all you need to solve this problem.

$$\sin 60° = a\,/\,g$$

$$\frac{\sqrt{3}}{2} = a\,/\,g$$

$$a = \frac{g}{2}$$

The wrong answer choices: Choice A should be eliminated because it expresses force, not acceleration. Choice C is a trap. You'd fall for it if you'd referred to an angle of 30° instead of 60°. Choice D is wrong, plain and simple.

53. When an electron is added to a neutral atom to form its anion, the atomic radius:

   A. decreases, because the added electron makes the orbital more complete.
   B. increases, because the effective nuclear charge decreases.
   C. increases, because the electronegativity of the atom decreases.
   D. stays the same, because the added electron contributes neglible mass to the atom.

53. **B** is correct. When you review periodic trends, you'll learn that atomic size reflects effective nuclear charge. The added electron will decrease effective nuclear charge, which will increase atomic radius.

The wrong answer choices: Choice A is wrong because the extra electron increases the total negative charge around the nucleus. The number of protons and the degree of positive charge are constant. Electrons are thus able to "spread out" and increase the atom's radius. Choices C and D make true statements at their core, but they don't explain the status of atomic size.

54. Two sinusoidal waves, one with a frequency of 14 cycles per minute, the other with a frequency of 12 cycles per minute, are sent down a rope. The frequency of the combined wave is:

   A. 14 cycles/min.
   B. 26 cycles/min.
   C. 84 cycles/min.
   D. 168 cycles/min.

54. **C** is correct. To answer this question, you find the least common multiple of 12 and 14:

   $12 = 2^2 \times 3^1$ and $14 = 2^1 \times 7^1$. Hence, the lowest common denominator:

   $2^2 \times 3^1 \times 7^1 = 84$.

(This question does not ask for the frequency of the *beat*, which is 2 cycles/minute.)

The wrong answer choices: B is a trap. You would add 14 and 12 only if they were measures of the relevant *amplitudes*. D is also a trap. Although 168 is a common multiple of 12 and 14, it isn't the *smallest* common multiple. A is *not* a trap. It's just wrong, plain and simple.

55. The atomic radius of $^{22}_{11}$Na is approximately twice that of $^{40}_{18}$Ar, mainly because:

A. the ionization energy of Ar is greater than that of Na.

B. Ar is inert, whereas Na easily forms an ion.

C. the valence electrons of Na are more effectively shielded from the nucleus than the valence electrons of Ar.

D. Ar has 18 protons attracting its electrons, whereas Na has only 11 protons.

55. C is correct. The question is about *effective nuclear charge,* and you'll be able to answer it after you review periodic trends. Within a period, movement from left to right normally corresponds to a decrease in atomic radius because additional protons "pull" on the outermost electrons. Once a shell is complete, however, the next added electron begins a *new* shell. The new shell is partially shielded from the protons by the complete shell lying "beneath." Hence, with the beginning of a *new shell*, there is a sudden *increase* in atomic radius.

The wrong answer choices: Choices A and B are wrong because ionization energy and chemical reactivity fail to explain the observed difference in atomic radii. Choice D makes a true statement but does not account for the facts that (1) Ar also has 18 *electrons* being pulled by its 18 protons, and (2) Na has 11 electrons for its 11 protons.

56. Approximately what is the period of the wave produced by the tuning fork?

   A. .0007 s
   B. .0023 s
   C. .0071 s
   D. .0440 s

56. B is correct. Your review of waves will remind you that period is the inverse of frequency:

$$T = 1/440 \text{ Hz} = .0023 \text{ s}$$

57. Which of the following figures best represents a standing sound wave inside the tube?

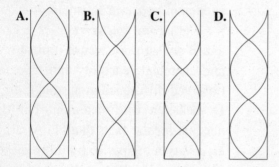

57. D is correct. The Princeton Review students know how to answer this question without referring to the passage. After studying basic wave properties, you'll know that waves are inverted when reflected from a fixed boundary and remain upright when reflected from an unfixed boundary. The closed end of the tube represents a fixed boundary, and the open end represents an unfixed boundary. That's why you should expect a node at the closed end of the tube and an antinode at the open end.

58. If the tube's diameter were increased, which of the following would be true regarding the period and/or frequency of the standing wave inside it?

   A. Its wavelength would increase.
   B. Its wavelength would decrease.
   C. Its period would increase.
   D. Its wavelength and period would remain unchanged.

58. D is correct. After your review of physics, you'll be able to answer this question by applying your knowledge of waves and using a simple process of elimination.

The wrong answer choices: Choices A and B are wrong because wavelength depends on the length of the tube, and velocity depends on the medium of travel. Neither factor relates in any way to the tube's diameter. Choice C should be eliminated as well. Period is simply the reciprocal of frequency and depends only on (1) the length of the tube and (2) the wave's velocity.

59. As the water level in the tube is lowered, resonance occurs at intervals of .37 m. This implies that the speed of sound in air is:

A. 163 m/s.
B. 326 m/s.
C. 330 m/s.
D. 370 m/s.

60. The room in which the experiment takes place is filled with helium. The density of helium gas is much less than that of air. What changes will occur to the standing wave?

A. The distance between antinodes will increase.
B. The distance between antinodes will decrease.
C. The distance between antinodes will remain the same.
D. No standing wave will form.

61. Which of the following would indicate that the tuning fork was rapidly moving away from the end of the tube?

A. The amplitude of the sound waves reaching the tube is greater than expected.
B. The amplitude of the sound waves reaching the tube is less than expected.
C. The frequency of the sound waves reaching the tube is greater than expected.
D. The frequency of the sound waves reaching the tube is less than expected.

59. B is correct. The pertinent information is provided in paragraph 1. Knowing that resonance occurs at odd quarters of the wavelength, you can conclude that:

$$(1/2) \lambda = .37 \text{ m}$$
$$\lambda = .74 \text{ m}$$

The frequency of the wave is provided to you:

$$v = \lambda \nu$$
$$v = (.74 \text{ m})(440 \text{ Hz})$$
$$v = (.74 \text{ m})(440^{-1})$$
$$v = 326 \text{ m/s}$$

The wrong answer choices: Choices A, C, and D are wrong. Choice A is a trap. You'd fall for it if you used .37 m for l. Choice C describes the speed of sound *in air*. Choice D is not a trap. It's just wrong, plain and simple.

60. A is correct. A medium's composition and density determine the speed at which it will facilitate the propagation of waves. Helium gas is less dense than air, so sound waves travel faster through helium than through air. You know that $v = \lambda \nu$; if v increases and ν remains the same, λ must increase. An increase in wavelength will appear as a separation of antinodes.

61. D is correct. Your review of waves will include a study of the Doppler effect. If a wave's source travels away from an observer, it will seem to the observer that the wave is longer than expected. Since frequency is the inverse of wavelength, increased wavelength corresponds to decreased frequency. The perception of "stretching" is only apparent when there is a basis for comparison, such as with a train whistle that approaches, then moves away from an observer. That basis of comparison is lacking in this example.

62. If the number of moles of a gas in a 1 liter container is decreased at 300 K, which of the following figures best represents the relationship between the number of moles and pressure?

A.

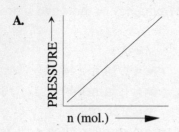

B.

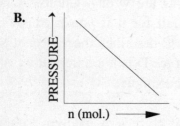

C.

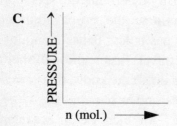

D.

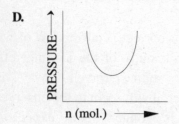

62. A is correct. Your chemistry review will naturally include a tour through the ideal gas law: $PV=nRT$. As the number of moles of gas decreases, pressure must decrease, and the correspondence is *linear*. Choice A reflects the appropriate relationship.

The wrong answer choices: Choice B is wrong because the indicated graph suggests that as the number of moles increases, the pressure decreases. Choices C and D should be eliminated because in relation to a sample of gas, you know that pressure is *directly proportional* to the associated number of moles. The appropriate graph must be linear and sloped.

63. A researcher wishes to compare real gas behavior to gas behavior predicted by the ideal gas law. The researcher subjects a gas sample to relatively high pressure and then compares the pressure actually measured to that which would be predicted according to the ideal gas law. The pressure *actually measured* is probably:

A. greater than that predicted by the ideal gas law because of repulsive forces among gas particles.

B. greater than that predicted by the ideal gas law because of attractive forces among gas particles.

C. less than that predicted by the ideal gas law because of repulsive forces among gas particles.

D. less than that predicted by the ideal gas law because of attractive forces among gas particles.

63. **D** is correct. When it comes to gas behavior, the MCAT requires that you appreciate this simple fact: ideal gas behavior is just that—*ideal*. It isn't real. Rather, it's based on two unrealistic assumptions: (1) that gas particles themselves have no volume, and (2) that gas particles do not attract one another. In fact gas particles (1) do have (very small) volume of their own and (2) attract one another via van der Waals forces, dipole interactions, and London dispersion forces. Such attractive forces are especially significant under conditions of high pressure and they result in real pressures that are *lower* than those one would predict by applying the ideal gas equation PV – nRT. That's why D is right.

The wrong answer choices: Choices A, B, and C are of the upside-down, inside-out variety. They're a smoke screen that keeps you from thinking clearly and selecting the correct answer. As you can see, each is wrong because it either replaces "greater" with "more," or "attractive" with "repulsive."

64. A decrease in the number of moles of a gas at constant temperature and volume will decrease which of the following unit measures?

A. Cubic centimeters
B. Number of atoms per cm^3
C. Joules per mole of gas
D. Cubic centimeters occupied by the gas

64. B is correct. This question tests your knowledge of units. Consider the equation: $PV = nRT$. If T, R, and V are fixed, and n is decreased, it is true that the number of moles of gas per fixed volume decreases. In other words, there is a decrease in the number of atoms per cm^3. P would also decrease, but the units for P, Atmosphere/cm^3, is not an answer choice.

The wrong answer choices: Choice A is wrong because it does not reflect a proportional measure. Choice C is wrong because the only gas-equation variable with an energy component is R, and that's *constant*. Choice D is wrong because *you're told* that volume is constant.

65. Which of the following will demonstrate a greater departure from the behavior of an ideal gas: hydrogen gas or helium gas?

A. Helium gas, because the van der Waals corrections are lower than for hydrogen.
B. Helium gas, because it is an inert gas.
C. Hydrogen gas, because the van der Waals corrections are greater than for helium.
D. Hydrogen gas, because hydrogen shows decreased intermolecular forces at higher pressures.

65. C is correct. Paragraph 3 describes the real-gas corrections made to pressure and volume. Pressure becomes $P + (an^2/V^2)$ and volume becomes $V - nb$, where a and b are constants characteristic of a particular gas. The table lists the values of a and b for He and H_2. Greater deviation from ideal gas behavior would correspond to greater values for a and b. The values of a and b are greater for hydrogen than for helium. That's why C is right.

66. Which of the following best illustrates the values of PV/RT in terms of pressure for hydrogen gas and a second gas, A_2, that shows greater compression at high pressures? (Note: The dotted line represents the values of PV/RT for an ideal gas under high pressures.)

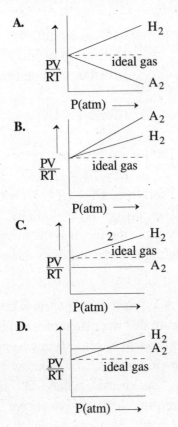

A.

$\frac{PV}{RT}$

P(atm) ⟶

H_2

ideal gas

A_2

B.

$\frac{PV}{RT}$

P(atm) ⟶

A_2

H_2

ideal gas

C.

$\frac{PV}{RT}$

P(atm) ⟶

2   H_2

ideal gas

A_2

D.

$\frac{PV}{RT}$

P(atm) ⟶

H_2

A_2

ideal gas

66. A is correct. Greater compression at higher pressures means that as pressure increases, there will be (1) a marked decrease in volume, V, and consequently (2) a decrease in the PV/RT ratio (since the numerator will be decreasing). Only Choice A's graph shows a decrease in the PV/RT ratio of gas A_2.

The wrong answer choices: Choice B should be eliminated immediately because it suggests that, as pressure increases, gas A_2 is unchanged or expanding. Choices C and D are wrong because they show A_2 behaving like an *ideal* gas, with the ratio PV/RT remaining constant.

67. From the passage above, what would be the van der Waals correction for the volume (cm³) for 2 moles of neon gas at pressures over 400 atm?

A. V - 0.02370
B. V - 0.0391
C. V - 2 × 0.02370
D. V - 2 × 0.0171

67. D is correct. The formula in paragraph 3 tells you that the corrected volume of a real gas is V-nb, where n represents the number of moles in the sample and b is a constant listed in the table. For 2 moles of neon, the corrected volume should be V-2(0.0171).

68. For an observer at point P viewing the image produced by the objective lens, the observer would see an image at:

A. $\dfrac{F}{4}$.

B. $\dfrac{F}{2}$.

C. the surface of the objective lens.

D. negative infinity.

68. D is correct. P is the focal point, which coincides with the focal length of this objective lens. To locate the image, we use the lens formula:

1/(focal length) =
1/(distance of image) +
1/(distance of object)

or, $1/f = 1/i + 1/O$

Then we substitute:
    $1/f = 1/i + 1/f$
Therefore, $1/i = 1/f - 1/f = 0$
The image is at infinity. By simple convention, the fact that the image appears to the left of the lens makes its distance *negative*.

69. Assuming that the incident parallel rays enter the objective lens at a small angle q to the axis of the telescope, which of the following figures shows a possible path for the light rays? (Some dimensions have been distorted for clarity.)

A.

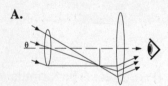

B.

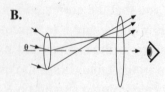

C.

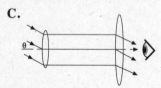

D.

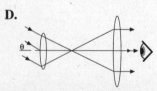

69. A is correct. You must take from the diagram this important piece of information: The objective lens is *converging*. After reviewing optics, you'll know that a ray is bent backward when it traverses a converging lens. It *converges* toward the focal point. If a ray enters the center of a converging lens it can't be bent at all. Choice A is consistent with these truths.

The wrong answer choices: Choices B, C, and D are wrong because they all show the ray bending as it enters the center of the lens.

70. With reference to the observer depicted in Figure 1, which of the following statements applies to the image at point P?

A. It serves as an object for the eyepiece.
B. It serves as an object for the objective lens.
C. It is real and upright.
D. It is virtual and inverted.

70. A is correct. The question requires that you have only (1) a certain comfort level with optical concepts and terminology and (2) an ability to comprehend the meaning of the passage. You are told that the "image at point P directs light rays to the eyepiece which transforms it into an enlarged virtual image. . . ." From the eye-piece's "point of view," in other words, the image at point P is an *object* that the eyepiece processes.

The wrong answer choices: Choice B is wrong because the question asks that you consider the situation from the observer's point of view. Light rays are traveling from left to right. Point P serves as object for the *eyepiece,* not as object for the objective lens. Choices C and D are wrong because, as you're told in the passage, the image at point P is *real and inverted.*

71. The two lenses in Figure 1 act together as a single equivalent lens with a focal length of:

A. $F + f$.
B. $F \times f$.
C. $\dfrac{Ff}{F + f}$.
D. $\dfrac{F + f}{Ff}$.

71. C is correct. The question is fully answerable without reference to the passage. A good review of optics will remind you that lens power, P, is the inverse of focal length: $P = 1/f$. It's also important to know that power is additive and that focal lengths are not. If two lenses act as one, their powers sum: Total power = $1/F + 1/f = 1/$(total focal length). Hence total focal length is correctly reflected in choice C.

The wrong answer choices: Choices A and B would be right only if focal lengths were not inversely additive. Choice D is a trap. You'd fall for it if you forgot to *invert* the total power to solve for total focal length.

72. If the observer is viewing a comet that is moving toward the telescope, how will the image seen by the observer differ from one of a stationary body?

A. The color of the image corresponds to that of a lower frequency.
B. The color of the image corresponds to that of a higher frequency.
C. The image will be brighter.
D. The image will be more blurred.

72. B is correct. The question does not draw on the passage. After studying sound and light, you'll realize that this question tests your understanding of the Doppler effect. As the source of sound or light waves moves toward a stationary observer, the frequency of perceived light or sound increases.

The wrong answer choices: Choice A is wrong because it describes the result of a comet moving *away* from the observer. Choice C is wrong because the comet would appear brighter only if the *intensity* of its emitted light increased. Choice D is wrong because the comet is so distant that the telescope is assumed to preserve focus: The image is never blurred.

73. Referring to the light rays drawn in Figure 1, which of the following is true?

A. The objective lens is a diverging lens.
B. The eyepiece lens is a diverging lens.
C. Both lenses are converging lenses.
D. Both lenses are diverging lenses.

73. C is correct. Figure 1 shows you that both lenses bend light inward toward a focal point. That means both lenses are converging.

The wrong answer choices: Choices A, B, and D are wrong because none of the lenses is diverging. In other words, none of them bends light rays *outward*.

Freestanding (Questions 74–77)

74. Based on the table below, which of the following species is the weakest oxidizing agent?

Half-Reaction	Standard Potential
$Br_2(l) + 2e^- \rightarrow 2Br^-(aq)$	1.08
$Ag_2O(s) + H_2O + 2e \rightarrow 2Ag(s) + 2OH^-(aq)$	0.34
$Cu^{2+}(aq) + e^- \rightarrow Cu^+(aq)$	0.15
$H_2(g) + 2e^- \rightarrow 2H^-(aq)$	0.00

A. H_2
B. Cu^{2+}
C. Br_2
D. Ag_2O

74. A is correct. When you take the MCAT and you're dealing with "redox" reactions, you think like this: A weak oxidizing agent means something that's: (1) *not* good at oxidizing things, (2) very willing to *be* oxidized, (3) *good* at reducing things, and (4) *not* very willing to *be* reduced. This question presents you with *reduction* half-reactions and the associated standard potentials. With that information you're supposed to figure out which of the named species is the weakest *oxidizing* agent. That means you're looking for something that's not very willing to be reduced, which means, in turn, that you're looking for the *lowest* standard reduction potential on the table. The lowest number on the table is 0, which means that among the species listed, H_2 is the weakest oxidizing agent. That's why A is right.

75. An atom is in its ground state with all the orbitals filled through n = 2 main energy level. How many electrons are contained in this atom?

A. 8
B. 10
C. 12
D. 14

75. B is correct. A quick way to count the electrons is to sketch the configuration that fills the second energy level:
$$1s^2 2s^2 2p^6; \ 2 + 2 + 6 = 10$$

76. A uranium-238 nucleus emits an alpha particle (helium nucleus) and decays to thorium-234. The alpha particle leaves the nucleus traveling 4.68×10^5 m/s. At what speed would the thorium nucleus recoil? (Note: Assume the masses of a proton and a neutron are equal.)

A. 1.5×10^3 m/s
B. 4.0×10^3 m/s
C. 8.0×10^3 m/s
D. 2.5×10^4 m/s

76. C is correct. This question asks only that you understand conservation of momentum.
$$m_1 v_1 = m_2 v_2$$
$$v_1 = m_2 v_2 / m_1$$
$$v_1 = (4 \text{ amu})(4.68 \times 10^5 \text{ m/s}) / (234 \text{ amu})$$
$$v_1 = 8 \times 10^3 \text{ m/s}$$

PHYSICAL SCIENCES EXPLANATIONS 165

77. The half-life of material X is 1 min. The half-life of material Y is three times greater than that of material X. Starting with 1 g samples of X and Y, how much more of material X would have decayed after 6 min?

A. $\dfrac{7}{32}$ g

B. $\dfrac{15}{64}$ g

C. $\dfrac{3}{8}$ g

D. 2 g

77. B is correct. In 6 minutes, X completes 6 half-lives. After 6 half-lives, 63/64 of material X is decayed. In 6 minutes, Y completes 2 half-lives. After 2 half-lives, 3/4 of material Y is decayed.

$$63/64 \text{ g} - 3/4 \text{ g} = 15/64 \text{ g}$$

WRITING SAMPLE EXPLANATIONS

The following essays were written according to The Princeton Review's MCAT Essay Formula. As described in Part I, they are designed to make a "good impression" on a reader who will spend approximately *ninety seconds* evaluating them. Notice that each essay:

- performs, in appropriate order, all three "tasks" described in the MCAT instructions,

- provides frequent paragraphing,

- uses formal language, and—

- cites a quotation from some famed authority.

WRITING SAMPLE EXAMPLE #1

People get the government they deserve.

Essay:

The statement indicates that in all societies people constitute the ultimate power, that they bear responsibility for their destiny, and that a government, however corrupt or abusive, reflects that which the people choose or tolerate. (The notion that people are generally responsible for their own fate is manifest also in Mohandas K. Gandhi's remark that "Good government is no substitute for self-government.")

If in a democracy a legislature or leader should fail to serve the people's interest, the people might be said to "deserve" the result because it is they who vote. Likewise, it might be argued that even a totalitarian dictator is incapable of installing *himself* in power. He must at some point have the active or passive approval of the citizenry.

In order specifically to describe a situation in which the statement does not apply, one need only recognize that the words "people" and "deserve" are inherently ambiguous. The statement pivots on these words, and its applicability depends on the meanings attached to them.

As used in the statement, "people" is subject to interpretation. No government comes to power with the unanimous approval of the populace, and in many situations, past and present, minority political groups have sought actively to overthrow a sitting government. It is unfair to suggest, for example, that occupied Europe's underground movements were in any way responsible for Nazi governance. Participants in such movements sought aggressively to defeat the Nazis, and in no sense can they be said to have "deserved" life under the occupying power even though they were *people* and for a time it *was* their government.

The word "deserve" also harbors ambiguity. If it carries some *moral* implication then it is proper to say that there are a great many situations to which the statement does not apply. The fact that a people should be ignorant, naive, or misguided does not mean that they are morally deficient or that in some moral sense they "deserve" a government hostile to their interests.

For example, during the 1988 presidential election campaign many Americans were misled by one candidate's promise of "no new taxes" and did not believe those who warned them that new taxes would be necessary regardless of who became president. When the candidate won, he broke his promise. Voters who were then disturbed by tax increases did not deserve their disappointment in the sense that they were bad or evil for believing that a candidate would keep his word.

Hence the pertinence of the statement depends in large measure on the meaning attached to its language. If "people" refers to the majority of the people, and if "deserve" refers only to the concept of responsibility, then perhaps the statement represents a meaningful comment. If however, "people" means *all* people and "deserve" imparts some moral justice, the statement is not a useful insight.

WRITING SAMPLE EXAMPLE #2

Honesty is essential to friendship.

Essay:
The statement indicates that a genuine bond of friendship requires truthfulness and that in its absence friendship is false. (The statement seems implicitly, also, to extol true friendship as Ben Jonson did when he wrote, "True happiness consists not in the multitude of friends but in the worth and choice.") The statement suggests that two people are not truly friends, for example, if they are unable to confide in one another or if one habitually deceives the other.

In order specifically to describe a situation in which the statement does not apply, one need only recognize that the words "honesty" and "friendship" are inherently ambiguous. The statement pivots on these words, and its applicability depends on the meanings attached to them.

As used in the statement, "honesty" is subject to interpretation. There is probably no person living or dead who has ever revealed to any other person all the details of every thought or experience he has ever had. It is doubtful that any person is capable of such openness. It probably is not fair to suggest that one who has difficulty sharing certain of his thoughts and feelings cannot have and cannot be a friend.

Furthermore, there are occasions on which total truthfulness between two persons would violate the confidence of a third. One who has been trusted with the secret of another in a personal or professional context is wrong to reveal it even to a true friend. One's friendship with another person is not impaired because he guards the secret of a third. Indeed, if that were not so, one could never have more than one friend.

The word "friendship" also harbors ambiguity. In some contexts the term simply describes social acquaintances. In others it imports deep, long-lasting, confidential relations. Social acquaintances can and do proceed on only small amounts of honesty. Hence when a "group of old high school friends" gets together for a reunion, it can scarcely be said that a high degree of personal honesty is essential to their interaction. Yet they still might call themselves "friends." Deep confidential relationships, on the other hand, do call for a significant commitment to truthfulness, and friendship conceived in that sense does require honesty.

Hence the pertinence of the statement depends in large measure on the meaning attached to its language. The statement represents a legitimate comment if "honesty" refers to a substantial commitment to truthfulness (with due regard for the rights of others) and if "friendship" refers to relatively deep and confidential relationships. If however, "honesty" means total candor in all respects and "friendship" denotes any and every relationship tagged with the label "friend," the statement does not furnish a useful insight.

BIOLOGICAL SCIENCE EXPLANATIONS

Passage I (Questions 1–6)

1. In humans, the peptide bonds of ingested proteins are first cleaved in the stomach by which of the following enzymes?

   A. Lactase
   B. Pepsin
   C. Amylase
   D. Lipase

1. **B is correct.** The question has nothing to do with the passage. To answer correctly you need only know this: pepsin is the gastric enzyme that cleaves peptide bonds.

   The wrong answer choices: After you've studied digestive enzymes, you'll know that choices A, C, and D are wrong because lactase, amylase, and lipase do not act on proteins, but on other substrates.

2. Colloid pressure tends to draw fluid into the blood vessels by:

   A. passive diffusion along a concentration gradient.
   B. passive diffusion along an electrical gradient.
   C. facilitated transport along an electrochemical gradient.
   D. active diffusion, mediated by an ATP-dependent pump.

2. **A is correct.** This question requires that you read paragraph 2. The protein concentration gradient between blood vessels and interstitial fluid produces passive diffusion.

   The wrong answer choices: Choice B is wrong because the gradient is not electrical. Choices C and D are wrong because in this case fluid movement depends on neither a carrier molecule nor the expenditure of energy.

3. A professor theorized that if a patient's capillaries became suddenly permeable to protein, the patient would manifest edema. Is this a plausible hypothesis?

   A. No, fluid will move across a membrane only in response to an ion gradient.
   B. No, protein permeability would have no effect on hydrostatic pressure within the blood vessel.
   C. Yes, protein would fuel the active transport of fluid into the interstitial space.
   D. Yes, colloid pressure would decrease, and fluid would leak into the interstitial space.

3. **D is correct.** You'll find the important information in paragraph 2. Protein in the interstitial space would draw water in an "attempt" to balance the colloid pressure.

   The wrong answer choices: Choices A and B should be eliminated because they present false statements. Why do we say that? Because fluid may move across a membrane in response to a number of influences. An ion gradient is only *one* such influence. Protein permeability will alter hydrostatic pressure within a blood vessel. Choice C is wild and unjustified.

4. The blood proteins that produce colloid pressure are synthesized by a sequential mechanism that involves the direct activity of:

A. cellular proteases.
B. smooth endoplasmic reticulum.
C. messenger RNA.
D. cytochromes.

4. **C** is correct. The question is unrelated to the passage. It draws on your knowledge of the fact that messenger RNA directs protein synthesis from amino acids.

The wrong answer choices: After studying cellular biology, you'll know that choices A, B, and D are wrong because none is associated with protein synthesis: Proteases degrade protein, smooth endoplasmic reticulum forms part of the intracellular membrane, and cytochromes are a part of the electron transport chain.

5. Given the results of Experiments 1 and 2, a researcher would be most justified in concluding that:

A. Cadaver D had a higher protein concentration in its interstitial fluid than did Cadavers A, B, or C.
B. Cadaver A contained more interstitial fluid than did Cadaver B which contained more interstitial fluid than did Cadaver C.
C. Cadavers A, B, and C were composed of at least 50 percent interstitial fluid by weight .
D. Cadaver C was composed of approximately 80 percent interstitial fluid by weight.

5. **C** is correct. The tables show that all three cadavers had a weight of at least 60 kg before infusion began and that all had a weight of less than 30 kg after 70 minutes. During the interim, interstitial fluid was removed from all cadavers. That means that all of the cadavers were originally composed of at least 50 percent interstitial fluid (because at least *half* of the total weight in fluid was drawn off from each of cadavers A, B, and C).

The wrong answer choices: Choices A, B, and D are wrong simply because there is nothing in the table that supports any of the statements they represent.

6. If, in a normal patient, proteins were suddenly infused into the interstitial space, which of the following physiological compensations could prevent the resulting edema?

A. Reduction of hydrostatic pressure within the blood vessels

B. Passive diffusion of proteins from the blood vessels to the interstitial space

C. Facilitated diffusion of protein from the blood vessels to the interstitial space

D. Increase in protein synthesis by the red blood cells

6. **A** is correct. Paragraph 2 explains hydrostatic force. Reduced hydrostatic pressure within the blood vessels decreases the fluid volume forced into the interstitial space.

The wrong answer choices: Choices B and C are wrong because paragraph 2 states that in a normal person blood vessels are impermeable to protein. That means neither passive nor facilitative diffusion will move protein from blood vessels to the interstitial fluid. Choice D is wrong because red blood cells do not directly regulate fluid balance between blood cells and interstitial space.

7. When concluding that the drop in oxygen consumption is due only to inhibition of cytochrome b, the researchers most probably assumed that Antimycin A:

A. increases levels of CO_2.
B. decreases levels of oxygen in the atmosphere.
C. attacks only the respiratory chain.
D. attacks other oxidative mitochondrial enzymes.

7. C is correct. This question tests experimental reasoning. Oxygen consumption might decrease for reasons unrelated to the respiratory chain. That means the researchers could fully attribute the decrease to cytochrome b inhibition only if they assumed that Antimycin A acted solely on the respiratory chain.

The wrong answer choices: Choice A makes a false statement. The assumption that Antimycin A increases carbon dioxide levels is not justified by the passage. Choice B makes a false statement because Antimycin A reduces oxygen consumption, so it wouldn't decrease levels of atmospheric oxygen. Choice D should be eliminated because the passage states that applying Antimycin A inhibits cyotchrome b.

8. Which of the following phosphorous-containing compounds can circumvent the effects of rotenone, as seen in Figure 1?

A. $FADH_2$ circumvents the effects of rotenone.
B. Both NADH and ADP circumvent the inhibition.
C. Both NADH and ADP circumvent the inhibition; $FADH_2$ also circumvents the effects of rotenone, but it does not contain phosphorous.
D. $FADH_2$, NADH, and ADP circumvent the inhibition of NADH dehydrogenase by rotenone.

8. A is correct. According to Figure 1, $FADH_2$ enters the respiratory chain *after* the step at which rotenone acts. Therefore, application of rotenone has no effect on the activity of $FADH_2$.

The wrong answer choices: Choices B and D make false statements. ADP enters the respiratory chain at the point where rotenone would effectively inhibit it, and NADH would be affected in the second step of the respiratory chain. Choice C also makes a false statement. ADP and NADH do not escape inhibition by rotenone, and $FADH_2$ contains phosphorous.

9. Aerobic organisms generate the greatest number of ATPs when monosaccharide oxidation produces:

   A. reduced levels of anti-oxidants.
   B. reduced forms of NAD⁺ and FAD.
   C. oxidized forms of ATP and GTP.
   D. oxidized forms of NADH and FADH₂.

9. **B** is correct. Paragraph 1 tells you that NADH and FADH$_2$ transfer electrons to produce ATP. NADH and FADH$_2$ can be referred to as reduced forms of NAD$^+$ and FAD. In other words, the reduced form of a molecule is associated with H$^+$ and has potential for greatest energy release.

The wrong answer choices: Choices A and C should be eliminated. They're wild and irrelevant. Choice D makes a false statement. Oxidized forms of NADH and FADH$_2$ correspond to NAD$^+$ and FAD. These molecules have already lost their H$^+$ and with it their potential for energy release.

10. A substance that inhibits NADH-Q reductase will have little effect if the cell is adequately supplied with which phosphorous-containing compound?

    A. FADH₂
    B. NADPH
    C. ADP
    D. NADH

10. **A** is correct. The diagram indicates that FADH$_2$ bypasses inhibition of NADH-Q reductase. That's because FADH$_2$ enters the respiratory chain *beyond* the site of NADH-Q reductase inhibition. (A blocked bridge won't stop you from reaching your destination if your route *doesn't cross the bridge*.)

The wrong answer choices: Choice B should be eliminated because NADPH is not a component of the respiratory chain. Choices C and D are wrong because NADH and ADP enter the respiratory chain "upstream" of the site at which NADH-Q reductase inhibition occurs.

11. The presence of fully functioning respiratory chains in the mitochondrial extracts was vital to the success of the experiment. If cytochrome c_1 had been missing, the researcher most likely would have found that:

A. extra cytochrome c_1 had accumulated.
B. NADH and $FADH_2$ could not enter the system.
C. Antimycin A had increased oxygen consumption.
D. Antimycin A had had no effect.

11. **D** is correct. Figure 1 shows you that Antimycin A blocks the step bridging cytochrome b and cytochrome c_1. If cytochrome c_1 were missing, then that step of the respiratory chain "connecting" cytochrome b to cytochrome c_1 would fail before exposure to Antimycin A.

The wrong answer choice: Choice A should be eliminated because it's wild. cytochrome c_1 is a component of the respiratory chain and does not vary in number in response to changes in other respiratory chain components. Choice B makes a false statement. Entry of NADH and $FADH_2$ into the respiratory chain is not affected by absence of cytochrome c_1 farther down the chain. Choice C makes also a false statement. The passage states that the effect of Antimycin A is to *decrease* oxygen consumption.

12. To further characterize cytochrome b, the researchers reacted its sulfur-containing amino acids with performic acid and then broke apart the polypeptide into individual amino acid residues. The most likely means of performing this latter task is to:

A. reduce cysteine residues.
B. decarboxylate acidic residues.
C. oxidize amide linkages.
D. hydrolyze amide linkages.

12. **D** is correct. After reviewing the biochemistry of cells, you'll know that a "peptide bond" is an "amide bond." (It's the amide bond that holds amino acids together to make proteins.) If one hydrolyzes peptide bonds, one is hydrolyzing amide bonds.

The wrong answer choices: Choice A should be eliminated. It's wild and irrelevant. Choice B makes a false statement. The process of breaking a polypeptide into its component amino acids does not involve decarboxylation. Choice C also makes a false statement. The breakage of an amide linkage occurs through *hydrolysis*, not oxidation.

13. The heme portions of cytochrome molecules are able to transfer electrons among themselves because of:

A. thioether linkages.
B. pi-electron delocalization.
C. enol-intermediate racemization.
D. shortened bond length.

13. **B** is correct. The question is unrelated to the passage. It requires that you review organic chemistry. Once you do, you'll know that the heme portions of cytochromes are characterized by pi-electron delocalization that stabilize the structure.

The wrong answer choices: Choice A makes a false statement. Thioethers are thiol derivatives and are not associated with heme resonance structure. Choice C also makes a false statement. An enol-intermediate represents one of the forms that carbonyl molecules assume. It is *not* associated with heme resonance structure. Choice D is wild and irrelevant.

Passage III (Questions 14–18)

14. Which of the following best describes the appearance of *Lactobacillus* when stained and then viewed with a light microscope?

  A. Spherical
  B. S-shaped
  C. Rodlike
  D. Asymmetrical

14. **C** is correct. There is nothing in the passage that helps you answer this question. You need only know that *Lactobacillus* belongs to the bacterial group "bacilli." After reviewing microbiology, you'll recall that bacilli are rod-shaped.

  The wrong answer choices: Choices A and B are wrong because spherically shaped and S-shaped bacteria describe the appearance of cocci and spirilli, respectively. Choice D is wrong because symmetry of form has no bearing on the classification of bacteria.

15. The proliferation of *Lactobacillus* in milk samples indicates:

  A. high lactose concentration.
  B. a drop in the pH.
  C. predominance of sporeforming bacteria.
  D. the absence of *Streptococcus faecalis*.

15. **B** is correct. Paragraph 1 describes the environmental conditions that promote growth of *Lactobacilli*. A reduced pH provides a receptive environment for Lactobacilli.

  The wrong answer choices: Choice A should be eliminated because it contradicts paragraph 1, which tells you that lactose must be converted to lactic acid to spur *Lactobacilli* growth. Choices C and D are wrong because in relation to the growth of *Lactobacillus*, the passage does not mention sporeforming bacteria or *Streptococcus faecalis*.

16. If one of the raw milk samples were heated to 100° C for 30 minutes, the graph of sporeforming and nonspore-forming bacteria would be which of the following?

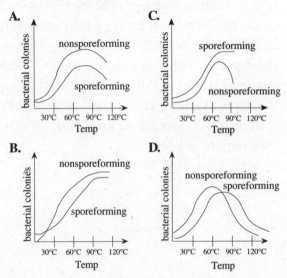

16. C is correct. The essential information is provided in paragraph 1. You're told that pasteurization kills nonsporeforming bacteria. You may infer that sporeforming bacteria are better able to resist the high temperatures of pasteurization.

The wrong answer choices: Choices A and B should be eliminated because the graphs they present indicate high survival rates for nonsporeforming bacteria that undergo pasteurization. Paragraph 1 states that nonsporeforming bacteria do *not* survive pasteurization. Choice D is wrong because it indicates that pasteurization kills sporeforming bacteria.

17. The gram-staining procedure used in the laboratory enables the inspector to:

   A. identify bacterial species present in the incubate.
   B. distinguish between aerobic and anaerobic organisms.
   C. differentiate pathogenic from nonpathogenic colonies.
   D. distinguish between bacterial and viral organisms.

17. A is correct. The question has nothing to do with the passage. It requires that you review microbiology and know that gram staining pertains to bacterial identification.

The wrong answer choices: Choices B and C are wrong because gram staining does not elucidate metabolic processes. Choice D should be eliminated because gram staining pertains to bacteria, not to viruses.

18. Which of the following environmental factors will affect the growth of *S. faecalis*?

  I.   Nutritional content of the milk
  II. The process of pasteurization
  III. Ambient oxygen concentration

A. I only
B. I and II
C. I and III
D. I, II, and III

18. **A** is correct. The important information is provided in paragraph 1. You're told that *S. faecalis* grows in milk, which contains emulsified fat droplets. Therefore, option I is correct. Option II makes a false statement because *S. faecalis* is a *spore-forming* bacteria. The passage states that pasteurization kills *non*sporeforming bacteria. Option III also makes a false statement. *S. faecalis* is *anaerobic*. It does not require oxygen.

Freestanding (Questions 19–24)

19. The *eclipsed* conformation of *n*-butane is illustrated below, in the figure on the left. Which of the circled positions in the figure on the right corresponds to the terminal methyl group in the *anti* conformation?

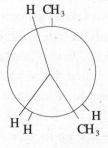
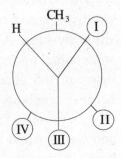

A. I
B. II
C. III
D. IV

19. C is correct. Butane has two methyl groups that rotate freely about the carbon-carbon single bond. When it comes to butane, the *eclipsed* conformation means that the methyl groups overlap. The *anti* conformation means the methyl groups are situated "across" from one another. With reference to the picture, the position that's directly across from the n=butane's methyl group is position III. That's why C is right.

20. All of the following structures secrete enzymes that serve digestive functions EXCEPT:

A. pancreas.
B. stomach.
C. thymus.
D. mouth.

20. C is correct. After reviewing mammalian physiology, you'll know that the thymus is a site at which lymphocytes mature.

The wrong answer choices: Choices A, B, and D are wrong because all of the named structures produce enzymes important to digestion. The pancreas secretes enzymes that decompose starch, protein, and fat. The stomach secretes pepsin, which digests protein. The mouth secretes amylase, which digests starch.

21. Alkyl halides are more reactive than their corresponding alkanes because the halides more readily participate in:

A. pyrolysis.
B. combustion reactions.
C. hydrophobic bonding.
D. nucleophilic substitution.

21. **D** is correct. Alkyl halides are more reactive than their corresponding alkanes because they all feature the functional group OH^-, which makes them readily susceptible to nucleophilic substitution. That's why D is right.

The wrong answer choices: Choice A is wrong because pyrolysis refers to decomposition by heat. Alkyl halides are no more susceptible to that sort of decomposition than are the alkanes. Choice B is wrong because combustion refers to reaction with oxygen (burning) to produce carbon dioxide and water. Alkyl halides are no more combustible than are their corresponding alkanes. Choice C is wrong because there is no such thing as "hydrophobic bonding."

22. When lettuce is placed in deionized water it remains crisp because:

A. the cells lose H_2O.
B. the cells swell with H_2O.
C. the stomates close in response to excess water.
D. the chloroplasts generate greater levels of ATP.

22. **B** is correct. After reviewing the biology of cell membranes, you'll know that a medium of pure water is hypotonic compared with a cell placed within it. Water will enter the cell in an "attempt" to balance the high solute concentration within the cell.

The wrong answer choices: Choice A is wrong for this reason: Water would leave the cell only if the cell's solute concentration were *lower* than that of its surrounding medium. Choice C is wrong because stomata tend to *open* in the presence of water. Choice D is wrong because chloroplast activity is irrelevant to the question.

23. Among the following, which statements can be said to apply to the hypothetical molecule depicted schematically below?

I. It rotates the plane of polarized light to the left
II. It exhibits chirality
III. It is optically active

A. I only
B. I and II
C. I and III
D. II and III

24. Which statement below most accurately describes the characteristic features of striated muscle cells?

A. Striated muscle cells are stimulated by the autonomic nervous system and contain few mitochondria.
B. Striated muscle cells are mononucleate and arranged in syncytial bundles.
C. Striated muscle cells have alternating A-bands and I-bands arranged in a transverse pattern.
D. Striated muscle cells are similar to smooth muscle cells except they lack internal stores of calcium.

23. D is correct. The hypothetical molecule reveals a carbon bonded to four distinct and different substituents. A carbon so situated constitutes a "chiral center" and the entire molecule itself is "chiral." A chiral molecule is optically active, which means that it rotates the plane of polarized light *either* to the right or left. However, one cannot ascertain the actual direction of rotation except by resorting to a polar-imeter or by knowing *a priori* the direction in which the molecule's enantiomer ("mirror image molecule") rotates polarized light. That's why options II and III apply and option I does not.

24. C is correct. After reviewing the musculo-skeletal system, you'll know that striated muscle cells contain "thick filaments" that correspond to the sarcomere's A-band and "thin filaments" that correspond to its I-band.

The wrong answer choices: Choice A is wrong because striated muscle cells are not stimulated by the *autonomic* nervous system. They're stimulated by the *somatic* nervous system. Choices B and D are wrong because striated muscle cells are multinucleate and are structurally dissimilar to smooth muscle cells (although both smooth and striated muscle cells store calcium).

Passage IV (Questions 25–29)

25. Which of the following treatments would NOT be an effective means of treating Candidal infections?

   A. Administration of a drug that attacks the outer cell wall of the fungus
   B. Administration of a drug that interferes with fungal replication and transcription
   C. Exposure to the infective form of the fungus itself
   D. Exposure to oral fungistatic drugs

26. Attacking the gamete-producing stage of Candida does NOT rid the body of Candidal infection because:

   A. the fungus does not reproduce by the formation of gametes.
   B. the fungus can be killed only by using drugs that also kill the host.
   C. the fungus produces gametes that are insensitive to all known drugs.
   D. the fungus is most often in a form that reproduces asexually.

27. 5-FC attacks the Candida fungus by decreasing:

   A. the need for formation of gametes.
   B. the availability of DNA and RNA precursors.
   C. the availability of necessary amino acids.
   D. the availability of 5-FU.

25. **C** is correct. This question requires some common sense. Exposure to the infective form of the fungus would make the infection worse.

The wrong answer choices: Choices A, B, and D represent false statements because each describes an *effective* treatment for Candidal infection.

26. **D** is correct. This question requires that you read paragraph 2, which tells you that Candida can divide asexually. Asexual reproduction involves *no* gametes. Therefore, one could *not* control the infection by attacking Candida's gamete-producing stage.

The wrong answer choices: Choice A is wrong because paragraph 2 tells you that Candida do produce gametes. Choices B and C should be eliminated because they represent false statements. Neither drug toxicity to the host nor the idea of a drug-insensitive gamete is mentioned in the passage.

27. **B** is correct. Paragraph 3 tells you that 5-FC leads to a decrease in thymidine formation. After reviewing molecular biology you'll know that thymidine is a precursor to *both* DNA and RNA.

The wrong answer choices: Choices A, C, and D are wrong. With reference to the effect of 5-FC, the passage does not mention gamete formation, amino acid availability, or 5-FU availability.

28. After absorption of 5-FC, which next step must occur for 5-FC to terminate DNA synthesis?

    A. One pyrimidine is substituted for another pyrimidine.

    B. A purine must be converted into a pyrimidine.

    C. Uracil must be converted into thymidine.

    D. Thymidylate synthetase must be phosphorylated to be inactivated.

28. A is correct. Paragraph 3 provides the important text. It tells you that Candida cells convert 5-FC to 5-FU. After reviewing cell biochemistry you'll know that both cytosine and uracil are pyrimidines.

The wrong answer choices: Choice B makes a false statement. 5-FC is not a purine. It's a pyrimidine. Choice C should be eliminated because it distorts the meaning of the passage. You're told that 5-FU *inhibits* production of thymidine. It doesn't *become* thymidine. Choice D should be eliminated too. With reference to thymidylate synthetase, phosphorylation and inactivation are not mentioned.

29. When undergoing reproduction, the predominant form of Candida in the human body according to the passage maintains:

    A. the same number of chromosomes per nucleus, while randomly dividing the genome between two daughter cells.

    B. the same number of chromosomes per nucleus, without randomly dividing the genome between two daughter cells.

    C. half the number of chromosomes per nucleus, without randomly dividing the genome between two daughter cells.

    D. half the number of chromosomes per nucleus, while randomly dividing the genome between two daughter cells.

29. B is correct. The pertinent text is in paragraph 2, which tells you that Candida divide primarily by asexual budding. After reviewing cell division, you'll recall that mitosis gives rise to *non*random division of the genome.

The wrong answer choices: Choice A makes a false statement. Asexual reproduction proceeds by mitosis. In the process of mitosis, genetic material is *not* divided randomly. Choice C also makes a false statement. Mitosis does not involve a halving of genetic material. Choice D represents *both* false statements set forth in choices A and C.

Passage V (Questions 30–36)

30. Which of the following ovarian cell organelles will show the greatest levels of activity during the secretion of estrogen steroids?

A. Lysosomes
B. Golgi apparatus
C. Plastids
D. Ribosomes

30. **B** is correct. The question is entirely unrelated to the passage. It requires that you review cellular biology so you can remember that the Golgi apparatus *packages* steroids (and other substances) destined for secretion. In an actively secreting cell, the Golgi apparatus is busy.

The wrong answer choices: Choice A makes a false statement. Lysosomes contain and degrade those of the cell's substances and structures that are "old and worn-out." Choice C is wrong because plastids are limited to plant cells. Choice D makes a false statement. Ribosomes are active in *protein* synthesis.

31. Which test groups showed the greatest levels of estrogen synthesis and secretion?

   I. Onset of menstruation
  II. Ovulation peak
 III. Pregnancy, 160 days
 IV. Pregnancy, term

A. I and III
B. I and IV
C. II and III
D. III and IV

31. **D** is correct. This question requires that you consider Table 1, keeping a particularly close watch over the relevant units. Look at the test groups labeled "pregnancy, 160 days" and "pregnancy, term." For these two groups, estrogen secretion is measured in mg. In all other test groups, estrogen level is measured in µg, a smaller unit. Once you're alerted to the units, you can see that the two named test groups do show the highest levels of estrogen synthesis and secretion. That's why options III and IV are correct.

32. From Table 1, which variable would prove to be the best marker for the term stage of normal pregnancy, as indicated by the Kober test?

    A. The oxidation of estradiol
    B. The presence of estriol
    C. The presence of 16a-hydroxyestrone
    D. A positive Kober reaction

32. C is correct. The question calls for some common sense. Table 1 shows you that 16a-hydroxyestrone appears only for the test group labeled "pregnancy, term." Hence, it would *tell you* that a patient is in the term stage of pregnancy. That's another way of saying 16a-hydroxyestrone acts as an *indicator* for the term stage of pregnancy.

The wrong answer choices: Choice A should be eliminated. With reference to the term stage of pregnancy, the passage does not mention estradiol oxidation. Choice B makes a false statement. Estriol is present in *all* test groups. Choice D also makes a false statement. A positive Kober test indicates only that estrogen is present, and estrogen is present in *all* test groups.

33. Would estrogen levels in males increase at the onset of puberty?

    A. Yes, because the increased levels of testosterone in the pubertal male are partially converted to estrogens.
    B. Yes, because the increased rate of respiration in pubertal males leads to a decrease in testosterone levels.
    C. No, because estrogen hormones are produced only by abnormal human males.
    D. No, because estrogen hormones do not vary in amount at the onset of puberty in the male.

33. A is correct. Your review of the endocrine system will remind you that males can convert testosterone to estrogen.

The wrong answer choices: Choices B and C should be eliminated. They're wild and irrelevant. Choice D makes a false statement because estrogen levels may vary at the onset of male puberty.

34. In Table 1, which of the following pairs of subject groups showed the greatest differences in the ratios of estrone to 16-epiestriol levels?

    A. Pregnancy/160 days and postmenopause
    B. Pregnancy/term and pregnancy/160 days
    C. Postmenopause and pregnancy/160 days
    D. Onset of menstruation and postmenopause

34. B is correct. Only one of the choices sets forth a ratio of estrone to 16-epiestriol levels. That's because only one choice considers the test group "pregnancy, term" — the only stage of the cycle at which 16-epiestriol appears.

35. What change in the ratio of estrone to estradiol is expected to occur as women enter postmenopause, according to the passage?

- **A.** The ratio increases, because estradiol levels decrease relatively more than estrone levels decrease.
- **B.** The ratio increases, because estradiol levels decrease while estrone levels are unaffected.
- **C.** The ratio is unchanged, because both estrogen hormone levels decrease in the postmenopausal period.
- **D.** The ratio decreases, because estrone levels decrease more than estradiol levels.

35. A is correct. Table 1 provides the important information. For premenopausal women, the ratio of estrone to estradiol levels is approximately 2:1. For postmenopausal women, it's about 4:1.

36. Researchers further studied estrogen levels in subjects at the luteal minimum of estrogen secretion and at the 210th day of pregnancy. Which findings would NOT indicate a trend similar to that found during the original procedures?

- **A.** The levels of estriol are greater than the levels of estradiol in both pregnant and luteal minimum groups.
- **B.** The levels of estradiol are lower than those of estrone in the pregnant group.
- **C.** The estrone levels are elevated in the pregnant group compared with the luteal minimum group.
- **D.** The ratio of 16-epiestriol levels between the pregnant and luteal minimum groups is 1:2.

36. D is correct. According to Table 1, 16-epiestriol appears *only* at the term stage of pregnancy and not at anything called the "luteal minimum stage." The study would contradict the data in the table.

The wrong answer choices: Choices A, B, and C are wrong because each of the named findings is fully consistent with the data set forth on Table 1.

Passage VI (Questions 37–42)

37. When alkyl halides react with potassium hydroxide to yield alkene derivatives, the potassium hydroxide acts as:

A. an acid.
B. a base.
C. a proton donor.
D. a reductant.

37. B is correct. Once you review elimination reactions, you'll recall that an alkene may be formed from an alkyl halide in the presence of a strong base, like OH⁻. Consider, for example, ethylchloride:

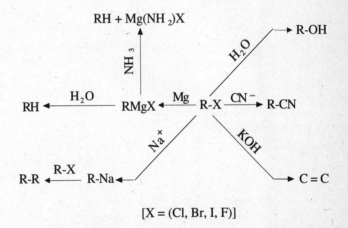

$$[X = (Cl, Br, I, F)]$$

The OH- removes a proton from the first carbon, leaving it with a lone pair of electrons. This lone pair then moves between the two carbons, where it forms a double bond and simultaneously removes the chloride atom from the second carbon.

The wrong answer choices: Choices A and C should be eliminated because OH- is not an acid and certainly cannot *donate* a proton. Choice D is wrong because the OH- does not *reduce* the carbon.

38. If one were to substitute heavy water in the last steps of the Grignard reagent, the reaction would lead to the synthesis of:

A. R-R.
B. R-OD.
C. R-D.
D. R-H.

38. C is correct. After you study alkyl halides and their reactions, you'll know that alkyl halides can react with water (undergo hydrolysis) to yield a hydrocarbon and a metal hydroxide. Remember that "heavy water" is designated: D_2O.

So, $RX + D_2O \longrightarrow RD + XOD$.

The wrong answer choices: Choice A should be eliminated since individual alkyl groups won't react with one another. Choice B is wrong because water's oxygen provides a *binding site* for the halide. The oxygen does not *replace* the halide or bond with the central carbon. You would also eliminate Choice D pretty quickly if you remembered that heavy water is D_2O and contains deuterium instead of hydrogen.

39. Alkyl halides are not usually prepared by direct halogenation of alkanes because:

A. alkanes are not very reactive compounds.
B. alkanes have low boiling points.
C. alkanes are desaturated by halogenation.
D. alkanes do not dissolve in polarized solutions.

39. A is correct. After you study the alkanes and their reactions, you'll know that alkanes are *not* terribly reactive. Direct halogenation of an alkane occurs only under special conditions of extremely high temperatures or in the presence of certain light wavelengths.

The wrong answer choices: Choice B makes a true statement, but it does not explain why direct halogenation is not generally used to prepare alkyl halides. Choice C is wrong because desaturation refers to the addition of multiple bonds. Alkanes don't have double bonds. Choice D makes a true statement, but, like Choice B, it fails to answer the question.

40. The synthesis of ethane from methyl bromide requires the addition of:

   A. Mg and H_2O.
   B. Mg and RCH_2Cl.
   C. Na^+ and RCH_2Cl.
   D. Na^+ and CH_3Br.

40. **A** is correct. The question requires that you refer to Figure 1. It shows that R-X becomes a Grignard reagent (RMgX) when Mg is added. When H_2O is added, the Grignard reagent is converted to an alkane.

The wrong answer choices: Choice B is wrong because a Grignard reagent does not react with an alkyl halide. Organometallic compounds like Grignard's reagent generally react with water, diatomic halogens, oxygen, or metal salts (MX) only. Figure 1 shows you that Choices C and D are wrong. Reaction of R-X with Na^+ and then with R-X produces an elongated alkane.

41. Alkyl halides are insoluble in water because:

   A. they are hydrophilic.
   B. they are ionic compounds.
   C. they are unable to form hydrogen bonds.
   D. they contain electron-withdrawing groups.

41. **C** is correct. This question is unrelated to the passage. It requires that you know something about hydrogen bonding, polarity, and their relationship to water solubility. Solubility in water *requires* polarity. If alkyl halides could form hydrogen bonds they would necessarily be polar and, hence, soluble in water.

The wrong answer choices: Choice A is wrong because hydrophilic *means* water-soluble. Choice B is wrong because alkyl halide bonds are generally covalent. Choice D makes a true statement, but it is irrelevant and unresponsive to the question.

42. Identification of alkyl halides is often based on all of the following physical properties EXCEPT:

A. boiling point.
B. density.
C. spectroscopy.
D. mass.

42. **D** is correct. Compounds do not have inherent mass. Any given *sample* of a compound has a mass. But there is no such thing as a "compound's mass." (Compounds do, of course, have density and specific gravity, but that is not the same as mass.)

The wrong answer choices: Choices A and B are wrong because alkanes do have boiling points and densities. When you review alkane chemistry you'll know that, and such properties are useful in identifying alkanes. Choice C is wrong because a spectrum of IR absorptions positively identifies the presence of the "R-X stretch."

Passage VII (Questions 43–48)

43. Which of the following would NOT account for elevated levels of insulin in the blood?

   A. Ingesting a heavy meal
   B. Injecting insulin at bedtime
   C. Arising after an all-night fast
   D. Breaking a fast

44. Which of the following individuals would have the highest levels of glucagon in the bloodstream?

   A. A man running in the last third of a marathon
   B. A pregnant woman after eating breakfast
   C. A bedridden patient two hours after a meal
   D. A child after eating dessert

43. **C** is correct. Paragraph 2 provides the important information. You're told that insulin is secreted into the bloodstream in response to high glucose levels. After a fast, glucose levels would be *low*, not high.

The wrong answer choices: Choices A and D are wrong because ingesting a meal or *breaking* a fast would increase blood glucose. The increased glucose concentration would precipitate insulin secretion. Choice B is wrong because an insulin injection would naturally elevate insulin blood levels.

44. **A** is correct. The important text is in paragraph 2 which states that glucagon secretion follows from low blood glucose levels. Exercising would tend to reduce blood glucose levels and hence trigger secretion of glucagon.

The wrong answer choices: Choices B, C, and D are all wrong because they describe situations in which individuals have eaten without accompanying exercise. Blood glucose would not tend to be low in any such case.

45. The administration of insulin in Experiment 2 is able to reverse hyperglycemia because:

  A. insulin inhibits glucose uptake by body cells.
  B. insulin enhances glucose uptake by body cells.
  C. glucagon production by the liver is inhibited by insulin.
  D. levels of intracellular glucose are reduced by insulin.

45. **B** is correct. Paragraph 2 tells you that insulin causes glucose to move from blood to cells. Insulin administration reverses hyperglyclemia because it removes glucose from the blood (and admits it to the cells).

The wrong answer choices: Choice A makes a false statement. The passage establishes that insulin *increases* uptake of glucose by body cells. Choice C also makes a false statement. Insulin reverses hyperglycemia by directly increasing cellular glucose uptake, not by inhibiting glucagon production. Choice D is wrong because insulin causes the body cells to experience *increased* glucose concentration.

46. From what information can a researcher conclude that insulin and glucagon are produced by two different types of pancreatic islet cells?

  A. Certain islet cells have secretory products similar to those secreted by nervous system cells.
  B. High blood glucose increases the activity of some islet cells, while low blood glucose increases the activity of different islet cell types.
  C. Insulin and glucagon have opposing actions in the body.
  D. Insulin and glucagon have different polypeptide chains.

46. **B** is correct. The passage tells you that *high* blood glucose concentration is associated with insulin secretion and *low* blood glucose concentration is associated with glucagon secretion. Once you realize that, the question itself, together with simple logic, tells you that the two hormones must arise from different cell types.

The wrong answer choices: Choice A is wild and irrelevant. Choices C and D make false statements. Neither provides evidence that insulin and glucagon arise from distinctly separate cell types.

47. Body cells can respond in vivo to exogenously administered insulin because insulin is a polypeptide that interacts with cells via:

A. a bilayer membrane that allows simple inward diffusion of insulin.
B. a bilayer membrane that allows endocytosis of insulin.
C. cell receptors that are activated in close association with insulin.
D. cell receptors that degrade insulin on contact.

47. **C** is correct. The question is unrelated to the passage. After reviewing the biology of cell membranes, you'll know that polypeptides cross cell membranes only with the participation of cell receptors.

The wrong answer choices: Choice A makes a false statement. Insulin cannot cross the cell membrane by simple diffusion. Choice B also makes a false statement. Endocytosis is a process through which cells take in extraordinarily large molecules and particulate matter. Choice D also represents a false statement. Insulin would *never* affect cell function if it were systematically degraded on contact with the cell membrane.

48. What happened to the levels of blood glucose in the blood after insulin administration in Experiment 1?

A. Glucose was moved primarily into the liver and not other body tissues.
B. Glucose was moved primarily into the kidneys, as in diabetes insipidus.
C. Glucose was moved into body cells because insulin prevented blood cell degradation of glucose.
D. Glucose was moved into body cells because insulin increased the cells' uptake of glucose.

48. **D** is correct. Paragraph 2 tells you that insulin promotes cellular glucose uptake. It's that simple.

The wrong answer choices: Choices A and B are wrong because neither the liver nor the kidneys selectively takes in glucose, and the passage does not indicate that they do. Choice C is wrong because insulin does not affect blood cell degradation of glucose.

Freestanding (Questions 49–53)

49. Bacteriophages are viruses that attack bacteria. They attach to the surface of a bacterium and inject their genetic material into the host. Bacteriophages differ from other living organisms because:

   A. they lack the means to replicate inside a host cell.
   B. they have only RNA and must utilize a host cell's machinery to generate DNA.
   C. they lack the cellular metabolic machinery found in both eukaryotic and prokaryotic organisms.
   D. they possess bounding membranes and internal organelles including ribosomes and vacuoles.

49. C is correct. Your review of microbiology will remind you that viruses do *not* possess all of the cellular machinery that facilitates independent existence. Viruses rely on "host cells" to provide them with the apparatus necessary to reproduction.

The wrong answer choices: Choices A and B are wrong because bacteriophages proliferate by replicating within a host cell. Their genetic material is DNA. Choice D should be eliminated because it represents a false statement. Bacteriophages do not possess the named organelles.

50. Consider the reaction below.

$$C_5H_5NH^+$$

$$CH_3CH_2CH_2OH \longrightarrow CH_3CH_2CHO$$

Which of the following observations about the infrared spectrum of the reaction mixture would indicate that the reaction shown above occurred?

   A. The appearance of a C=O stretch and C–H stretch
   B. The appearance of an aliphatic C–H stretch
   C. The appearance of an O–H stretch
   D. The disappearance of an N–H stretch

50. A is correct. The compound on the left is an alcohol and the compound on the right is an aldehyde. Once you review infrared and nuclear magnetic resonance spectroscopy, you'll know that *infrared* spectroscopy would reveal the *disappearance* of the -OH group and the *appearance* of the C=O and C-H groups.

The wrong answer choices: Choice B is wrong because neither the reactant nor the product represents an aliphatic compound. Choice C is wrong because the O-H stretch will *dis*appear. Choice D is wrong because nitrogen does not belong to either the product or reactant.

51. The process of respiration consists of both inspiration and expiration. Inspiration is:

A. a passive process due to negative pressure in the thoracic cavity.

B. a passive process due to positive pressure in the thoracic cavity.

C. an active process due to negative pressure in the thoracic cavity.

D. an active process due to positive pressure in the thoracic cavity.

51. **C** is correct. Once you review respiratory physiology, you'll remember that inspiration is active and that it follows from the negative pressure that's created when the diaphragm contracts.

52. Sickle cell anemia is a blood disorder due to a point mutation in a single gene. It is inherited as an autosomal recessive trait. A woman is heterozygous for the disorder, having one normal allele on the genome and one allele affected by the point mutation. She most likely has:

A. full-blown sickle cell anemia.

B. sickle cell trait, a carrier disease.

C. no signs or symptoms of the disease.

D. a predominance of sickle-shaped red blood cells.

52. **B** is correct. An individual with sickle cell *trait* (as opposed to full-blown sickle cell disease) has certain adverse symptoms associated with sickled blood cells, but she does not have fulminant sickle cell anemia.

The wrong answer choices: Choices A and D are wrong because the woman *carrying* sickle cell trait has one normal allele which tends to produce red blood cells of normal shape. Choice C is wrong because the woman carrying sickle cell trait has one allele, which tends to produce sickle-shaped blood cells.

53. Which of the following is NOT a resonance structure of phenol?

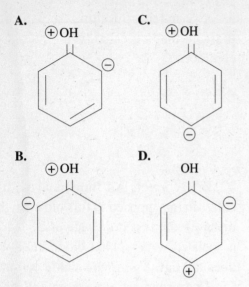

A.

C.

B.

D.

53. **D** is correct. When you review the chemistry of benzene, you'll know that benzene and its derivatives are "resonating" molecules. Benzene itself is a six-carbon ring with three double bonds dispersed about the ring. With reference to benzene, "resonance" refers to the dispersion of the double bonds. A simple *phenol* is benzene with an OH group attached to one of the ring carbons. The attachment of the OH group eliminates one of the ring double bonds. The ring's two *remaining* double bonds continue to be dispersed throughout the ring. A drawing will correctly depict a phenol resonance structure only if it shows both bonds distributed about the ring with charge appropriately assigned. Choice D is correct because it shows only one double bond within the ring and thus *fails* accurately to represent a phenol.

Passage VIII (Questions 54–58)

54. High total serum cholesterol puts a patient at risk for myocardial infarction because it reflects:

   A. low blood content of high-density lipoproteins.
   B. low blood content of low-density lipoproteins.
   C. high blood content of high-density lipoproteins.
   D. high blood content of low-density lipoproteins.

54. **D** is correct. Paragraphs 3 and 6 contain the important information. Together they tell you that low-density lipoprotein, the particle most associated with heart attack, makes up 60 to 70 percent of serum cholesterol.

   The wrong answer choices: Choices A and C are wrong because paragraph 4 tells you that high-density lipoproteins create no risk of myocardial infarction. Choice B is wrong because as stated in the passage, cholesterol is composed largely of LDL.

55. If an elderly woman with abnormally high levels of LDL has little coronary atherosclerosis, she most likely:

   A. has high levels of HDL, counteracting the effects of the LDL.
   B. follows a diet that is low in cholesterol-containing foods.
   C. has no atherosclerosis in arteries outside the heart.
   D. has failed to undergo a complete diagnostic screening for blood lipid status.

55. **A** is correct. The important information is in paragraph 4, in which you're told that a high *ratio* of LDL to HDL is associated with high risk of atherosclerosis.

   The wrong answer choices: Choice B should be eliminated because it represents a false implication. A low-cholesterol diet would explain low levels of LDL. It would not explain the absence of atherosclerosis in the face of high LDL levels. Choices C and D should be eliminated because they represent unwarranted conclusions.

56. Coronary atherosclerosis constitutes a medical problem because it threatens to:

A. render the heart less sensitive to stress.
B. produce imbalance in the patient's blood lipid profile.
C. compromise the heart muscle's oxygen supply.
D. subject the patient to high blood pressure.

56. C is correct. In paragraph 1 you learn that coronary atherosclerosis involves an accumulation of plaques within the coronary arteries. After you review the heart's anatomy, you'll know that the coronary arteries give the heart its blood supply. Since blood is the medium through which all tissues derive oxygen, any impairment of blood supply also compromises *oxygen* supply.

The wrong answer choices: Choices A and D should be eliminated because they distort the meaning of the passage. In paragraph 1 you're told that high blood pressure and stress may increase the risk of heart attack. You're *not* told that atherosclerosis causes high blood pressure or stress. Choice B also distorts the passage's meaning. In paragraph 1 you learn that a distorted blood lipid profile might lead to atherosclerosis. You *don't* learn that atherosclerosis leads to the distorted profile.

57. Coronary atherosclerosis is virtually unknown among peoples living in non-industrialized nations. This indicates that in comparison with industrialized populations these peoples probably have:

A. a lower incidence of heart attack.
B. a lower incidence of hypertension.
C. higher levels of VLDL.
D. higher levels of IDL.

57. A is correct. Paragraph 1 has the information you need. It tells you that coronary atherosclerosis is the leading cause of heart attack. Absence of atherosclerosis implies that fewer heart attacks will occur.

The wrong answer choices: Choice B should be eliminated because the passage makes no reference to the effect of athero-sclerosis on blood pressure. Choices C and D should be eliminated because the passage states that LDL and HDL affect the risk of atherosclerosis and heart attack. It makes no such statement about VLDL or IDL.

58. If coronary atherosclerosis produces myocardial infarction, what is the status of the affected heart muscle?

    A. High pH
    B. Low pH
    C. High O_2 concentration
    D. Low CO_2 concentration

58. **B** is correct. After reviewing the biochemistry associated with respiration and circulation, you'll know that low blood supply leads to increased metabolic waste formation. Metabolic waste (principally CO_2) in turn, produces acid (principally H_2CO_3). That, of course, *reduces* pH.

The wrong answer choices: Choice A is wrong because, as just explained, increased waste production *lowers* pH. Choices C and D are wrong because the decreased blood supply produced by atherosclerosis would impair *delivery* of oxygen and *removal* of carbon dioxide to and from the affected heart muscle.

Passage IX (Questions 59–65)

59. In studying the passage, one could estimate a dicarboxylic acid's K_1 value by determining:

   A. its concentration in a non-equilibrium mixture.
   B. its stability in anion form.
   C. its tendency to undergo decarboxylation.
   D. its crystallization structure.

59. B is correct. When you deal with chemical equilibria, you must remember: The more stable the products, the more likely it is that the reaction will proceed to completion. This means that K_1 is determined by the *relative stabilities* of a dicarboxylic acid's protonated and deprotonated forms.

The wrong answer choices: Choices A, C, and D are wrong because none of the named factors characterizes or influences equilibrium. As stated in the passage, equilibrium is characterized by the *ratio of products to reactants.*

60. Glutaric acid is a dicarboxylic acid with formula $HOOC(CH_2)_3COOH$. This acid is most likely to have a K_1 constant closest in value to which substance listed in the table?

   A. Fumaric acid
   B. Maleic acid
   C. Succinic acid
   D. Oxalic acid

60. C is correct. If you know that K_1 values decrease with increased number of double bonds, you'll realize that you should be looking for a compound whose structure is similar to that of glutaric acid. Among the choices, glutaric acid's molecular formula is most like that of succcinic acid. (Glutaric acid has one more (CH_2) group than does succinic acid.)

61. If equal concentrations of succinic acid, malonic acid, and maleic acid were heated in a weakly basic solution, which of the following products would be in the greatest concentration at equilibrium?

A. $HOOCCH_2COO^-$
B. $HOOC(CH_2)_2COO^-$
C. *trans*-HOOCCH=CHCOOH
D. HOOC-COOH

61. A is correct. The question requires that you understand, to some degree, the meaning of K_1 and that you read the table provided in the passage. Among succinic, malonic, and maleic acids, maleic has the highest K_1. That means its *de*protonated form will predominate. However, maleic is *not* among the answer choices. The next highest K_1 value is associated with malonic acid. That's why A is correct.

The wrong answer choices: Choice B is wrong because it represents the deprotonated form of succinic acid, which has a lower K_1 than does malonic acid. Choices C and D are wrong because they represent the protonated form of fumaric acid and oxalic acid, neither of which is present in solution.

62. In applying the information in the passage, it would be difficult to estimate K_1 for a molecule with the formula $HOOCCH_2NHCOOH$ because:

A. its anion stability is not directly comparable to that of succinic acid.
B. it cannot exist in the deprotonated form.
C. it must form an insoluble compound.
D. it represents an unstable compound.

62. A is correct. The anion of the indicated compound is not directly comparable to any structure listed on the table for the simple reason that *it contains an N-H group.*

63. In an aqueous mixture of maleic and fumaric acid, the equilibrium proportions can best be determined by which method?

A. Radioactive tagging of the corresponding alkene
B. Hydration of the anion solution
C. Acidification of the solution
D. Nuclear magnetic resonance spectroscopy of the equilibrium solution

63. D is correct. After you study NMR spectroscopy, you'll know that it is well suited to differentiate between *cis* and *trans* configurations.

The wrong answer choices: Answer choices A, B, and C are wrong for the simple reason that none of the named processes distinguishes between *cis* and *trans* configurations.

64. The value of K_1 of the dicarboxylic compound glutamic acid is substantially lower than the K_1 of glutaric acid because:

    A. glutamate is readily convertible into a nonpolar Zwitterion.
    B. glutamate's deprotonated form is less stable than the glutarate anion.
    C. glutamate is an amino acid.
    D. glutamic acid is a stronger acid than glutaric acid.

64. **B** is correct. From the passage you learn that lower K_1 value indicates a relatively lower tendency to deprotonate. After you study equilibria phenomena and acid-base organic chemistry, you'll know that the tendency to deprotonate, in turn, is a function of anion stability. Glutamic acid has a K_1 substantially lower than that of glutaric acid, which means that its anion is less stable than that of glutaric acid.

    The wrong answer choices: Choices A, C, and D are all wrong because, quite simply, the phenomena to which they refer are totally irrelevant to the question.

65. One can most reasonably estimate the value of K_2 for acetic acid (CH_3COOH) to be:

    A. higher than K_1 for acetic acid.
    B. higher than K_2 for maleic acid.
    C. lower than K_2 for oxalic acid.
    D. less than zero.

65. **C** is correct. A strategic reading of the passage teaches you that K_2 reflects a molecule's willingness to undergo double deprotonation. Once you review carboxylic acids, you'll know that acetic acid is a *mono*carboxylic acid, and that a monocarboxylic acid is most "unwilling" to undergo a second deprotonation. Oxalic acid is a *di*carboxylic acid that will much more readily undergo double deprotonation. Hence, the K_2 for acetic acid will naturally be lower than the K_2 for oxalic acid.

66. If a segment of the denatured viral DNA strand had a base sequence ATAA, what would have been the complementary RNA sequence?

A. GTGG
B. TATT
C. UAUU
D. TUTT

66. C is correct. The question has nothing to do with the passage. Your review of cell biochemistry will remind you of this: In the process of DNA-RNA transcription, a DNA adenine residue pairs with an RNA uracil residue. A DNA thymine residue pairs with an RNA adenine residue.

The wrong answer choices: Choices A, B, and D should be eliminated quickly because RNA never contains thymine. (It contains uracil instead.)

67. At the end of Experiment 3, how many offspring reproduced through the formation of gametes?

A. 0
B. 2
C. 4
D. 12

67. A is correct. The descriptions of Experiments 2 and 3 set forth the important information. You're told that reproduction occurred *asexually*. Asexual reproduction does not involve gametes.

The wrong answer choices: Choices B, C, and D are wrong because *none* of the organisms at issue underwent any form of sexual reproduction.

68. Suppose the lower-density Light strand mutant in Figure 1 cannot undergo transcription. The most likely explanation is that it does not:

A. bind DNA.
B. bind RNA.
C. bind protein.
D. replicate.

68. B is correct. The description of Experiment 1 provides the important information. You're told that the lower-density Light strand is viral DNA. The process of transcription requires that an RNA molecule align itself with a molecule of DNA. The Light strand's failure to undergo transcription means that the DNA cannot bind to RNA.

The wrong answer choices: Choices A and C are wrong because transcription requires that DNA bind to *RNA*, not to DNA or to protein. Choice D is wrong because transcription does not require DNA replication.

69. Mutated viral DNA Light strand produces no abnormal phenotypic changes, which is most likely due to the fact that the viral DNA Light strand:

   A. does not undergo translation.
   B. does not undergo replication.
   C. is contained in the nucleus.
   D. is able to undergo translation.

70. On what finding could one base the conclusion that the viral DNA Heavy strand normally produces transcribed mRNA, whereas the viral DNA Light strand does not?

   A. Neither the Heavy strand nor the Light strand of viral DNA can excise point mutations.
   B. Neither the Heavy strand nor the Light strand of viral DNA hybridizes with labeled RNA.
   C. Only mutated viral DNA Heavy strands exist in the natural setting.
   D. Only the mutated viral DNA Heavy strand produces phenotypic changes.

69. **A** is correct. The question is answerable without reference to the passage. After reviewing molecular cell biology, you'll know that proteins arise from translation and that they produce phenotypic traits. If transcription does not occur, proteins are not produced, and phenotypic changes do not result.

The wrong answer choices: Choice B is wrong because replication does *not* produce phenotypic change. Choice C is wild and irrelevant. Choice D is wrong because translation *can* produce phenotypic changes because it is important to the synthesis of proteins.

70. **D** is correct. The question has nothing to do with the passage. Transcription produces mRNA, which produces protein, and protein gives rise to phenotype.

The wrong answer choices: Choices A and B should be eliminated because neither describes a *distinction* between the Light and Heavy viral DNA strands. Choice C is wrong because it makes a false (and somewhat nonsensical) statement.

71. How can one conclude that mutations of the viral DNA Light strand do not affect phenotypic expression in the host?

A. By locating the mutation on the host DNA
B. By comparing Light strand mutants to Heavy strand mutants
C. By comparing the mutant phenotype with the unmutated form
D. By studying the production of RNA polymerase

71. **C** is correct. The question is unrelated to the passage. Instead, it requires simple common sense. In order to determine that mutation does or does not affect phenotype, one must simply *compare* the mutant and unmutated phenotype.

The wrong answer choices: Choice A is wrong because a mutation's location does not, of itself, indicate whether it will alter the host phenotype. Choice B is wrong because it describes the wrong comparison. The comparison should be between mutated and unmutated phenotypes. Choice D is wild and irrelevant.

72. By studying Figures 1 and 2, a scientist decided that the normal bacteriophage SP8 DNA consists of a double-stranded chromosome. For this conclusion to be true, which of the following assumptions must be correct?

A. Hybridization of DNA with RNA involves the formation of covalent bonds.
B. Radio-labeling affects the size of the RNA-DNA hybrid produced.
C. Mutation does not lead to changes in DNA sequence.
D. Denaturation breaks apart the double helix without hydrolyzing covalently attached base pairs.

72. **D** is correct. The question requires that you read Figure 2 strategically. The appearance of two peaks suggests the existence of two strands. That, in turn, indicates that the double-stranded chromosome separated without losing the covalently bonded base pairs on each strand.

The wrong answer choices: Choices A, B, and C are all wild and irrelevant.

73. For bacteriophage SP8, if the mutated Heavy strand codes for a protein that destroys DNA polymerases while the Light strand does not, then the mutant will:

A. show increased production of DNA.
B. show decreased evolutionary "fitness" compared with the Light strand mutant.
C. show increased evolutionary "fitness" compared with the normal virus.
D. show an increased tendency to undergo meiosis.

73. **B** is correct. The question is answerable without reference to the passage. It requires that you remember the meaning of evolutionary "fitness." If the Heavy strand mutant loses its DNA polymerase, *its ability to reproduce is impaired*, which means it's less "fit" than the Light strand mutant.

The wrong answer choices: Choices A and C make false statements. The defective heavy strand would experience *decreased* production of DNA and, hence, show *decreased* evolutionary fitness. Choice D should be eliminated because it's wild and irrelevant.

Freestanding (Questions 74–77)

74. Which of the following processes does NOT occur on the ribosomes during protein synthesis?

    A. Translation of mRNA
    B. Peptide bond formation
    C. Attachment of tRNA anticodons to mRNA codons
    D. Attachment of mRNA anticodons to tRNA codons

74. **D** is correct. After you study cell biochemistry, you'll remember that protein synthesis begins when transfer RNA (tRNA) "anticodons" align themselves with the codons of messenger RNA (mRNA). Choice D has it backward.

The wrong answer choices: Choices A, B, and C are wrong because each of the named processes does play a role in protein synthesis. Messenger RNA is fashioned on a DNA template. Peptide bonds are the "glue" that holds a protein molecule together, and transfer RNA anticodons carry amino acids, in appropriate sequence, to corresponding messenger RNA codons.

75. During embryonic gastrulation, invagination occurs as a result of which of the following processes?

    A. Release of a hormone
    B. Migration of cells
    C. Reproduction of cells
    D. Asymmetric division of cells

75. **B** is correct. After studying developmental biology, you'll know that in the process of gastrulation, cells *adjust their relative positions* to create three distinct germ layers (ectoderm, mesoderm, and endoderm).

The wrong answer choices: Choice A is wrong because hormones do not (as far as the MCAT is concerned) play any role in invaginating the blastula. C and D are wrong because cell migration, not cell *reproduction*, is the event that characterizes gastrulation.

76. Surgically implanted pacemakers are frequently used in the treatment of heart disease. Which of the following normal heart structures carries out the same function as a pacemaker?

A. The bundle of His
B. The atrio-ventricular node
C. The sino-atrial node
D. The sino-ventricular node

77. The hormone that most directly stimulates the formation of sperm in the testes is which of the following?

A. Estrogen
B. Testosterone
C. Luteinizing hormone
D. Follicle-stimulating hormone

76. C is correct. Your review of mammalian physiology will tell you that the sino-atrial node generates the heartbeat and is thus known as the heart's natural "pacemaker."

The wrong answer choices: Choices A and B represent false statements because each of the named structures fulfills functions other than pacemaking. The bundle of His conveys the heartbeat's electrical impulse outward along the walls of the ventricles. The atrioventricular node conducts it from atria to ventricles. Choice D is wrong because there is no such thing as the sino-ventricular node.

77. B is correct. After reviewing the endocrine system you'll know that sperm production requires testosterone.

The wrong answer choices: Choice A is wrong because estrogen does not play a role in sperm production. Choices C and D represent false statements. Luteinizing hormone and Follicle-stimulating hormone are indirectly related to sperm production. The two substances *regulate* testosterone secretion.

IF YOU NEED MORE SPACE, PLEASE CONTINUE ON THE BACK OF THIS PAGE.

TEST SHEETS 211

IF YOU NEED MORE SPACE, PLEASE CONTINUE ON THE BACK OF THIS PAGE.

212 CRACKING THE MCAT

STOP HERE FOR PART 1.

2 2 2 2 2

IF YOU NEED MORE SPACE, PLEASE CONTINUE ON THE BACK OF THIS PAGE.

214 CRACKING THE MCAT

IF YOU NEED MORE SPACE, PLEASE CONTINUE ON THE BACK OF THIS PAGE.

TEST SHEETS 215

STOP HERE FOR PART 2. DO NOT RETURN TO PART 1.

The Princeton Review
Diagnostic Test Form ○ Side 1

Completely darken bubbles with a No. 2 pencil. If you make a mistake, be sure to erase mark completely. Erase all stray marks.

1.
YOUR NAME: _____
(Print) Last / First / M.I.

SIGNATURE: _____   DATE: __/__/__

HOME ADDRESS: _____
(Print) Number and Street

City / State / Zip Code

PHONE NO.: _____
(Print)

IMPORTANT: Please fill in these boxes exactly as shown on the back cover of your test book.

2. TEST FORM

6. DATE OF BIRTH

MONTH	DAY	YEAR
○ JAN		
○ FEB		
○ MAR		
○ APR		
○ MAY		
○ JUN		
○ JUL		
○ AUG		
○ SEP		
○ OCT		
○ NOV		
○ DEC		

3. TEST CODE

4. REGISTRATION NUMBER

7. SEX
○ MALE
○ FEMALE

SCANTRON® FORM NO. F-592-KIN
© SCANTRON CORPORATION 1989 3289-C553-5 4 3 2
ALL RIGHTS RESERVED.

5. YOUR NAME

First 4 letters of last name / FIRST INIT / MID INIT

Begin with number 1 for each new section of the test. Leave blank any extra answer spaces.

SECTION 1

(Answer bubbles 1–100, options A B C D E)

The Princeton Review
Diagnostic Test Form ○ Side 2

Begin with number 1 for each new section of the test. Leave blank any extra answer spaces.

SECTION 2

SECTION 3

FOR TPR USE ONLY

V1	V2	V3	V4	M1	M2	M3	M4	M5	M6	M7	M8

NOTES

NOTES

NOTES

NOTES

ABOUT THE AUTHOR

Theodore Silver holds a medical degree from the Yale University School of Medicine, a bachelor's degree from Yale University and, in addition, a law degree from the University of Connecticut.

Dr. Silver has been intensely involved in the field of education, testing, and test preparation since 1976 and has written several books and computer tutorials pertaining to those fields. He became affiliated with The Princeton Review in 1988 and is chief author and architect of The Princton Review MCAT preparatory course.

Dr. Silver is Associate Professor of Law at Touro College Jacob D. Fuchsberg Law Center where he teaches the law of medical practice and malpractice, contracts, and federal income taxation.

THE PRINCETON REVIEW NETWORK

The Princeton Review wants to provide you with the most up-to-date information you need whether you are preparing to take a test or apply to school. If you are using our books outside of the United States and have questions or comments, or simply want more information on our courses and the services The Princeton Review offers, please contact one of the following offices nearest to you.

- HONG KONG   852-517-3016
- JAPAN (Tokyo)   8133-463-1343
- KOREA (Seoul)   822-795-3028
- MEXICO CITY   011-525-358-0855
- PAKISTAN (Lahore) 92-42-872-315
- SAUDI ARABIA   413-548-6849 (a U.S. based number)
- SPAIN (Madrid)   341-446-5541
- TAIWAN (Taipei)   886-27511293

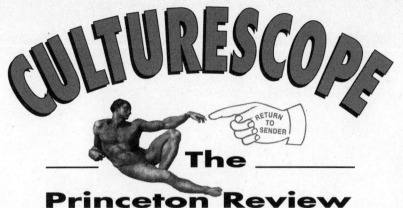
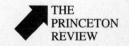